CW00586556

**The Acupuncture Role i**

Samir Yousef Ahmed AbouHussein

# The Acupuncture Role in Treatment of Diabetic Peripheral Neuropathy

## An Evidence-Based Literature Review Using a Novel Quality Assessment Tool

LAP LAMBERT Academic Publishing

**Imprint**

Any brand names and product names mentioned in this book are subject to trademark, brand or patent protection and are trademarks or registered trademarks of their respective holders. The use of brand names, product names, common names, trade names, product descriptions etc. even without a particular marking in this work is in no way to be construed to mean that such names may be regarded as unrestricted in respect of trademark and brand protection legislation and could thus be used by anyone.

Cover image: www.ingimage.com

Publisher:
LAP LAMBERT Academic Publishing
is a trademark of
International Book Market Service Ltd., member of OmniScriptum Publishing Group
17 Meldrum Street, Beau Bassin 71504, Mauritius

Printed at: see last page
**ISBN: 978-613-9-47225-3**

Zugl. / Approved by: Malta, University of Malta, Dissertation, 2017

**The Acupuncture Role in Treatment of Diabetic Peripheral Neuropathy**

An evidence-based literature review

**Samir Yousef Ahmed Mohamed Ali AbouHussein**
**M.D. (MBBS)**

**Supervisors**: Professor. Charles Savona Ventura (UM).
Professor Zhao Ling (SHUTCM).

*I would like to dedicate this work to my late parents (my beloved father, Alhag: Yousef and my beloved mother, Alhaga: Fatma) for shaping me to be the person I am today and for whom I cannot show my appreciation enough. They are always beloved and missed. I would also like to dedicate this work to all my family members [my great brother Mohamed, my niece Fatma, my great and sweet sister Monira, my brothers: Adel, Ali and Abdulla, and my sweet daughters (Wafa and Yasmeen) for their great love, support and encouragement.*

# Acknowledgements

The process of completing this Master degree course in Traditional Chinese Medicine and Culture program at the University of Malta in collaboration with Shanghai University of Traditional Chinese Medicine has been a highly challenging one, especially the completion of this capstone project. All the people who have been on this challenging journey with me have been kind, enthusiastic, supportive and generous with their time, expert advice and academic guidance. So, I would like to thank a group of people that helped me throughout this project.

I would like to thank my local supervisor; Prof. Charles Savona Ventura for his indispensable precious academic help and support throughout this course, and specifically for imparted his knowledge and wisdom throughout the process of preparing this literature review research.

Thanks are due also to my external supervisor Professor Zhao Ling from Shanghai University of Traditional Chinese Medicine for providing me with a number of Chinese literatures related to my dissertation which is very much appreciated and for his valuable suggestions about my prospective proposal

I would like to thank also to Prof. Sheng Liu from Shanghai University of Traditional Chinese Medicine for his great help in getting me some critically needed full articles of trials included in my study

I would like also to thank all the academic staff of University of Malta who enriched us with their high knowledge and professional expertise about the related study subjects of western medicine to Traditional Chinese Medicine

My thanks and gratitude are also due to all the academic staff from Shanghai University of Traditional Chinese Medicine who came all the way to teach us and give us the needed skills of various aspects of Traditional Chinese Medicine in highly qualified manner . These are; Prof. Ms. Qu Lifang, Dr. Ms. Fu Jingjing, Prof. Ms. Ke Cheng, Dr. Ms.Wang Fan, Prof. Mr. Yong Xia and Prof. Mr. Sheng Liu.

My ultimate credits go to all my family members as well as to my friend Mr. Leonard Godfrey Cassar for their inspiring moments in my life and for being so patient and showing me support, love and encouragement in many ways.

I sincerely appreciate you all and thank you from the depth of my heart for all your great love, support and patience throughout this process. Definitely all of you would be remembered fondly.

---

**Samir Yousef Ahmed Mohamed Ali AbouHussein**

# Abstract

**Back ground:** Diabetes mellitus is a global epidemic and in Malta, about 13.9% of the adult population is affected .The diabetic peripheral sensorimotor polyneuropathy is the most common Diabetic complication with the estimated prevalence in the range of 6.95%-9.73% in the Maltese population where the pharmaceutical therapy has very limited effect with high potential of side effects.

**Objectives:** To assess the clinical effectiveness and safety of acupuncture treatment for the management of diabetic peripheral neuropathy (DPN) as an add on complimentary treatment

**Methodology:** A total of about thirteen databases were systemically researched the period of the last 11 years (2006-2017). Total population of 1070 was included. The new modified quality assessment tool STRICTA Plus Score Scale (STRICTA-P) was used in this study to assess the quality of methodology design and reporting of the included RCTs. RCTs with score of >9 and active control treatments such as sham acupuncture or medical therapy were included. Out of a total of 63 potentially relevant articles which were retrieved in this literature review study, eventually, sixteen studies met the inclusion criteria and included in the actual assessment and the final analysis. Research language was limited to English; however reviews in Chinese were included and translated.

**Results:** The total efficacy rates in acupuncture treatment groups ranged from 83.33% to 95%. The average STRICTA-P score was 16.31 (74.15%), with FEI Ai-hua, et al 2011 has the minimum STRICTA-P of 12 (54.55%) and Garrow AP., et al 2014 has the maximum STRICTA-P of 19 (86.36%). Nevertheless, dissecting the STRICTA-P, shows that all the included trials failed to achieve 50% rate of the five points Jadad score (Jadad score ranged from 20% to 40%). Furthermore, 87.5% of the included trials scored zero for the Practitioner background score of (1) and only one study (Garrow AP., et al 2014) scored 1 (100%) and another study (Zhang C., et al, 2010) scored 0.5 (50%). However, the other scoring parameters of the novel STRICTA-P tool were relatively on average well scored in the included reviews.

**Conclusion:** This literature review showed that acupuncture treatment might be useful, effective and potentially safe complementary therapeutic tool in the management of DPN. However, these positive finding should be interpreted cautiously and conservatively, due to the fact that all included trials have high risks of bias. The heterogeneity of the included trials prevents us making a firm conclusion. The robustness of the results of the included trials could not be determined due to the fact that the majority of the included trials were of 'inadequate methodology' and low study population with multiple methodological and reporting biases. To ensure evidence-based clinical practice, further rigorous sham placebo-controlled, randomized trials are critically needed. These prospective trials need to be large scale studies and fully compliant with the CONSORT, STRICTA statements as well as the new quality assessment tool used in this study (STRICTA-P) to ensure high power and robustness as well as the clinical implications of their results.

**Key words:** Acupuncture, Diabetic Peripheral Neuropathy, DPN, Quality assessment tool, STRICTA, STRICTA PLUS Scoring Scale.

# Contents

# Figures List

## Tables List

# Abbreviations

| | |
|---|---|
| AA | Acupuncture analgesia |
| Ach | Acetylcholine |
| ADA | American Diabetes Association |
| AGE | Advanced Glycation End-products |
| AR | Aldose Reductase |
| ARI | Aldose Reductase Inhibitors |
| ATP | Adenosine Tri Phosphate |
| BL | Urinary Bladder Meridian |
| BP | Blood Pressure |
| CCK-8 | Cholecystokinin-octopeptide |
| COX-2 | Cyclooxygenase -2 |
| CRFs | Case Report Forms |
| CV | Conception vessel merdian |
| DAG | Di Acyl Glycerol |
| DD | Dense-Disperse |
| DNIC | Diffuse Noxious Inhibitory Controls |
| DPN | Diabetic Peripheral Neuropathies |
| DRG | Dorsal Root Ganglia |
| EA | Electro Acupuncture |
| EMG | Electromyography |
| EPC | Endothelial precursor cells |
| ERK | Extracellular signal-regulated kinase |
| EQ-5D | EuroQol 5-Dimension questionnaire |
| GB | Gall Bladder meridian |
| GV | Great Vessel meridian |
| HF | High Frequency stimulation |
| HRQoL | Health-Related Quality of Life |
| hs-CRP | hypersensitive C-reactive protein |
| Hz | Hertz |
| Inos | inducible Nitric Oxide Synthase |
| IGT | Intolerant to Glucose Test |
| IRRC | Institutional Research Review Committee |
| ITT | Intention-To-Treat analysis |
| KD | Kidney Meridian |
| LANSS | Leeds Assessment of Neuropathic Symptoms and Signs Scale |
| LDF | Laser Doppler fluxmetry |
| LF | Low frequency stimulation |
| LI | Large Intestine meridian |
| LOCF | Last Observation Carried Forward Analysis. |
| LR | Liver meridian |
| MA | Manual Acupuncture |
| MAPK | MAPK  Mitogen Activated Protein kinase |
| MCs | Mast Cells |
| MNCV | Motor Nerve Conduction Velocity |
| MYMOP | Measure Yourself Medical Outcome Profile |
| NADPH | Nicotinamide Adenine Dinucleotide Phosphate |
| NCS | Nerve Conduction Studies |
| NCV | Nerve Conduction Velocity |
| NDS | Neuropathy Disability Score |
| NGF | Nerve Growth Factor |

| | |
|---|---|
| NTSS-6 | Neuropathy Total Symptom Scale |
| NRS | Numerical Rating Scale |
| PP | Per-Protocol analysis. |
| PGP | Protein Gene Product |
| PKC | Protein kinase C |
| RCTs | Randomized Clinical Trials |
| ROS | Reactive Oxygen Species. |
| SA | Sham Acupuncture (SA) |
| SCI | Science Citation Index. |
| SDH | Sorbitol Dehydrogenase |
| SF 36 HS | Short Form 36 Health Survey |
| SJ | Sanjiao Meridian |
| SNCV | Sensory Nerve Conduction Velocity |
| SP | Spleen meridian |
| SPS | Sleep Problem Scale |
| SSR | Sympathetic skin responses |
| ST | Stomach meridian |
| STRICTA | STandards for Reporting Intervention in Controlled Trials of Acupuncture |
| STRICTA-P | STRICTA Plus Scoring Scale |
| STZ | Streptozotocin |
| TCM | **Traditional Chinese Medicine** |
| T2DM | Type 2 Diabetes Mellitus |
| T1DM | Type 1 Diabetes Mellitus |
| VAS | Visual Analogue Scale |
| WHO | World Health Organization |
| 5-HT | 5-Hydroxytryptamine |

# CHAPTER 1
# Introduction

## 1.0 Introduction

Diabetes mellitus is a global epidemic in developing and developed countries with estimated global sufferers of **366 million** by 2030.In Malta, there are currently about 44,100 cases of diabetes of the population which reflects an estimated prevalence of 13.9% of Diabetes in Adults in Malta [1].

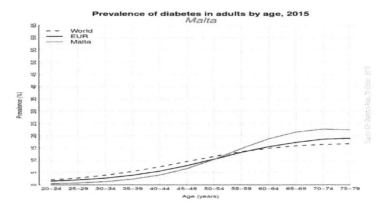

**Figure1.1: Prevalence of Diabetes in Malta in adults by age (adopted from Diabetes Atlas -7th Edition 2015).**

Diabetic Peripheral Neuropathies (DPN) are among the most common of all long-term micro-vascular complications of diabetes as it affects 50-70% of patients with diabetes [2-4]. The risk of having DPN increases with age and the duration of the diabetes (Figure1.1).

An International Consensus Meeting on the outpatient diagnosis and management DPN defined diabetic neuropathy as the presence of symptoms and/or signs of peripheral nerve dysfunction in people with diabetes after the exclusion of other causes [5].

2

## 1.1 Anatomical structure and vascular supply of peripheral nervous system:

The anatomical structural features of the peripheral nervous system might explain why the pathogenesis of neuropathy is distinct from other diabetic microvascular complications [6-8]. Few transperineurial arterioles penetrate through the perineurium covering peripheral nerves into the endoneurium (Figure 1.2). This causes the vascular supply of the peripheral nerves to be sparse so that blood flow is likely to be compromised and lacking auto-regulation [9]. This system makes peripheral nerves vulnerable to ischemia. The endoneurial microvessels are also tightly connected with endothelial cells on their inner surface, but when destroyed they are leaky and affect the endoneurial tissue components [10]. The leaky micro-vessels are mainly located in the ganglion with fenestrated vessels, and nerve terminals on the distal side are directly exposed to environments not covered by perineurium and are susceptible to traumatic injury. In Diabetes, the innervation of epineurial microvessels is involved, resulting in impaired blood supply in diabetic nerves [11, 12].


Histopathological tests illustrate that the endoneurial microvessels show thickened and multilayered basement membranes, cell debris of pericytes, as well as disrupted endothelial cells, and thus constitute salient structural changes in diabetic nerves [6]. Regardless of the vascular supply, the three dimensions of neuronal architecture specific to the peripheral nervous system might account for the reason why the most distal side is susceptible in diabetes. Ganglion cells have extensively long axons covered by Schwann cells. The neuronal cell body is relatively small compared with the extremely long distance of axonal neurites, and thereby distal axons are innately too weak to support themselves for the long transport of nutrients, nerve trophic factors, as well as other signals.

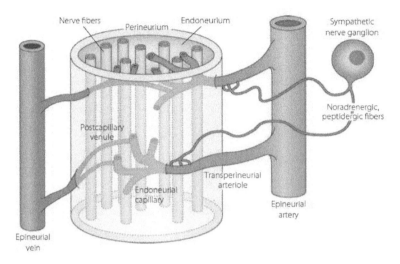

**Figure1.2: Vascular supply of the peripheral nervous system is sparse and transperineurial arteriole penetrates into endoneurium [Adapted from reference6].**

Although the autonomic nerve endings contact with the wall of arterioles, however, vascular auto regulation is lacking in peripheral nerves because of sparse innervations. In diabetes, autonomic nerve endings to the arteriole are likely to be lost and therefore vaso regulation is further impaired [6]. Subdivisions of sensory neurons are shown in Table1.1 and their correspondent classified nerve fiber endings are illustrated in Figure 1.3.

**Table1.1: Subdivisions of Sensory Neurons.**

| Fiber Type | Size | Modality | Myelination |
|---|---|---|---|
| A-alpha (I) | 13-20 micrometers | Limb proprioception | Yes |
| A-beta (II) | 6-12 micrometers | Limb proprioception, vibration, pressure | Yes |
| A-delta (III) | 1-5 micrometers | Mechanical sharp pain | Yes |
| C (IV) | 0.2-1.5 micrometers | Thermal pain, mechanical burning pain | No |

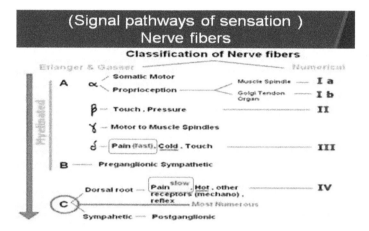

**Figure1.3: Sensory Nerve fibers subdivision with the correspondent sensation signal pathways (adapted from course lecture).**

## 1.2.0 Background Pathology of DPN

The patho-physiology of DPN remains unclear, although it is associated with increased age, duration of diabetes, lipotoxicity and glucotoxicity, genetic susceptibility, inflammation, and oxidative stress [13, 14].The most characteristic findings of the peripheral nervous system in diabetic patients are distal and sensory predominant nerve fiber degeneration, axonal loss and endoneurial microangiopathy [15, 16]. Both large and small caliber sizes of nerve fibers are affected. Dyck et al. 1986, proposed that microvascular injury is the most likely factor for focal fiber loss and its summation effect appears to be the cause of diffuse fiber loss of distal predominant axonal neuropathy in diabetes [17, 18]. However, a report showed that the focality of nerve fiber loss was not always demonstrated which might indicate that microangiopathy does not always account for the fiber loss [19]. Nevertheless, further studies on humans have been done to validate the vascular impact on the development DPN. Malik et al. 2003 has showed that patients who did not have clinically evident neuropathy at the time of nerve biopsy, but they demonstrated high-grade microangiopathic changes of endoneurial microvessels later, had developed overt neuropathy, whereas those without microvessel changes did not develop neuropathy [20].The degree of microangiopathic changes correlated well with the subsequent nerve fiber loss in diabetic nerves [21]. The most distal axons of small fibers distribute in the epidermis of the skin, sensing pain or pricking. Nowadays, punched skin biopsy immune-stained with protein gene product (PGP) - 9.5 is commonly used for the assessment of peripheral neuropathy [22].This method is minimally invasive, however it requires the equipment of confocal laser scan microscopy as well as skills for the staining and measurement. Generally, the skin over the calf muscle is used, but other sites could be added as well. In diabetes, the nerve fibers in the epidermis of the skin are significantly affected, resulting in twisting, distortion, focal swelling or beading, and eventually, loss of nerve fibers [23–25] (Figure 1.4).

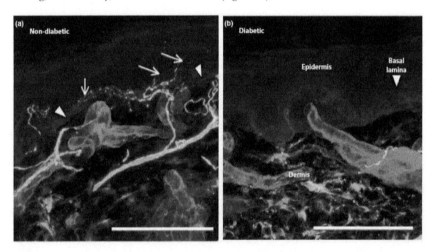

**Figure1.4: Epidermal innervations in diabetic patients as shown by immunostaining with PGP9.5.(a) In a normal subject-small branching fibers (arrows) penetrating to basal lamina (arrowhead) derived from dermis distribute diffusely and end in the surface of the epidermis of the skin. (b) In contrast, in a type 2 diabetic subjects with symptomatic neuropathy (with 15 years duration of diabetes), fibers in the epidermis are completely lost. Only a few fibers are sparsely left in the dermis. Vascular systems also develop in the upper dermis (red color of tortuous structure). Bar 100 mm(Adapted from reference [6]).**

In relation to the alteration of epidermal innervation, a non-invasive technique using corneal confocal microscopy has now been developed for the assessment of neuropathy [6, 26]. With this method, small nerve fibers distributed in the cornea can be observed without any need to tissue sampling in live conditions [27, 28]. Diabetic patients showed significant loss of nerve fibers, twisting and increased branching on the cornea [27, 28]. Considering the non-invasiveness nature of this technique, so, it is easy to follow by repeated observations and to evaluate the treatment effects on neuropathy by this method. Actually, the recovery of nerve fibers by regeneration was detected in long-standing type 1 diabetic patients 6 months after pancreas transplantation [29].

**How does hyperglycemia lead to peripheral nerve injury?**

Although, the etiology of diabetic neuropathy remains poorly understood, however, it has been proposed that persistent hyperglycemia can induce downstream metabolic cascades which will result in the peripheral nerve injury. The potential underlying mechanisms include;

➢ An increased flux through the polyol pathway,

➢ Glycation and advanced glycation end-products,

➢ Oxidative stress,

➢ Activation of protein kinase C and

➢ Pro-inflammatory processes [6].

The peripheral nerve injury to small unmyelinated C-fibers is initiated in the early stages of diabetes [30] and the hyperactivity of these fibers results in diabetic neuropathic pain [31]. Therefore, early detection of this impairment is suggested to prevent exacerbation of neurological complications and reduce severe pain symptoms [32].

## 1.2.1 The Polyol pathway

Increased polyol flux regulated by aldose reductase (AR) activation has been extensively studied and it has been demonstrated without doubt that this metabolic cascade contributes to the development of DPN. Accordingly, numerous AR inhibitors (ARI) have been developed, but clinical trials have largely been unsuccessful, in part due to the adverse effects or insignificant improvement at the clinical end-point. Currently, epalrestat is the only inhibitor licensed in Japan. It was approved after a 3-month double-blinded trial [33], which demonstrated reduction of symptoms and improvement nerve function. Further extended 3-year double-blinded randomized trials confirmed that ARI treatment significantly reduced the progressive delay of nerve conduction [34].The ARI effects were more marked in patients with early neuropathy and with modestly elevated levels of glycated hemoglobin [35].Another challenge of a new ARI will be expected to succeed in future trials, because other mechanisms do not amply replace the polyol pathway hypothesis [36, 37].

Despite a long history of preclinical studies, the detailed mechanism of how the polyol pathway is involved in neuropathy remains elusive. Earlier studies proposed the osmotic theory in which increased polyol flux caused intracellular hyperosmolarity by an accumulation of impermeable sorbitol in the cytoplasm, resulting in the expansion of cells and cell lysis [38, 39]. Although this theory might be applied to the genesis of diabetic cataracts [38, 39], there is no consistent evidence of nerve edema or swollen cells in diabetic nerve tissues [40]. Following the osmotic hypothesis, Greene raised the poor energy utilization theory as the surrogate of osmotic theory [41, 42]. With an accumulation of sorbitol, other osmolytes of myo-inositol, taurine and adenosine were reduced in the cytoplasm. In turn, myo-inositol deficiency caused phosphatidyl-inositol depletion and then poor production of adenosine triphosphate (ATP), leading to reduced activities of both; Na, K ATPase and protein kinase C (PKC) [41, 42]. However, there is no confirmative data of myo-inositol depletion in diabetic nerves [43]. Furthermore, clinical application of myo-inositol was not successful [44].

Consistent with the data from human intolerant to glucose test (IGT) subjects, it was shown that ob/ob mice revealed neuropathic changes represented by Nerve Conduction Velocity (NCV) delay and increased oxidative stress-induced damage [45]. High-fat diet fed mice that showed typical glucose intolerance also showed neuropathic changes [46]. In these mice, postprandial hyperglycemia itself exerted increased flux of the polyol pathway in the peripheral nerve tissues. The advent of transgenic technology has greatly advanced the polyol pathway story. Transgenic mice that over express human AR, developed severe neuropathy when they were fed galactose, which is also the substrate of AR [47]. Thus, without hyperglycemia or insulin deficiency, increased flux of the polyol pathway in fact caused peripheral nerve dysfunction and myelinated fiber pathology, similar to those found in diabetic animal models [47]. In addition to that; severe NCV delay and reduced Na,K-ATPase activity were observed with an accumulation of sorbitol and fructose, compared with those in non-transgenic diabetic mice, despite comparable levels of hyperglycemia[48]. The functional changes were accompanied by more severe structural changes in peripheral nerves and alterations of neuropeptide expressions in dorsal root ganglia (DRG) [49].The neuropathic changes were improved by giving diabetic transgenic mice ARI. In the contrary, studies that had used mice lacking the AR gene demonstrated that the AR-deficient mice were protective against neuropathy through the preservation of glutathione and nicotinamide adenine dinucleotide phosphate (NADPH) [50]. Although these studies have proved the significant role of AR in diabetic neuropathy, clinical experience of ARI trials [33] showed that the polyol pathway cannot fully explain the development of DPN because when blood glucose is poorly controlled, severe hyperglycemia can cause neuropathic changes, even in AR-deficient diabetic mice [51].

A pathway independent of AR is yet to be determined and further studies are required for the complete prevention or intervention of the progression of diabetic neuropathy. The implications of AR in ischemia/reperfusion injury have now revitalized the polyol pathway theory for vascular events are applicable, not only in diabetic patients but also non-diabetic patients (Figure 1.5). Ischemia/reperfusion causes polyol activation, leading to severe tissue injury against which ARI is preventive [52-58].Because diabetic nerves are susceptible to ischemia/reperfusion injury, a new perspective has been emerged that ischemia/reperfusion might be involved in the progression or exacerbation of neuropathy to which ARI is effective [59, 60]. Major regulating enzymes of the polyol pathway are differentially expressed in the epineurial artery and endoneurial tissues. Aldose reductase (AR) is strongly expressed in both the endoneurium and the wall of the epineurial artery, whereas expression of sorbitol dehydrogenase (SDH) is equivocal in the endoneurium, but clearly positive for the wall of the epineurial artery [61].

Figure1.5 illustrates the enhanced in situ expression of aldose reductase in peripheral nerve and renal glomeruli in diabetic patients. In contrast, the second portion of the polyol pathway regulated by SDH is activated in the vascular wall in the hyperglycemic condition. Then the enhanced synthesis of diacylglycerol (DAG) results in increased protein kinase C (PKC) activity. Yamagishi et al 2003 study demonstrated that major PKC isoforms which underwent changes in the diabetic condition are PKCa (α-isoform)in the nerve and PKCb (β- isoform)in the epineurial artery) [62].

Recently, a new role of aldose reductase in ischemia/reperfusion and inflammatory injury was proposed. When a cell becomes ischemic, glucose uptake is augmented to compensate energy depletion. Consequently, free radical injury and PKC activation ensue to aggravate ischemic injury. Once reperfusion starts, oxygen radicals accumulate aldehydes, which are also substrates of aldose reductase, and enhance radical injury (Figure 1.6).

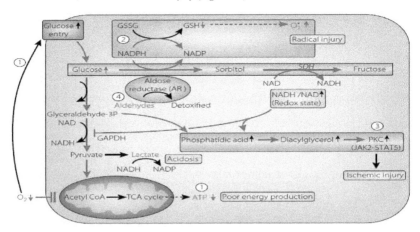

**Figure1.5: The implication of aldose reductase in ischemia/reperfusion injury (Adapted from reference 6).**

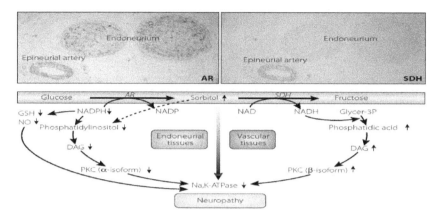

**Figure1.6: Tissue-specific regulation of polyol pathway and its metabolic cascade to diabetic neuropathy (Adapted from reference 6).**

## 1.2.2 The Glycation and the Advanced Glycation End-products

Glycation has long been implicated in the pathogenesis of diabetic neuropathy [63-65]. The deposition of advanced glycation end-products (AGE) was shown in human and animal diabetic nerves, in every component of peripheral nerve tissues [63, 65]. The degree of AGE deposition was well correlated with reduced density of the myelinated nerve fiber [66]. Several nerve tissues, such as Schwann cells, nerve fibers and endothelial cells of vasa nervosum all express receptor for AGE (RAGE) [6]. Figure1.7 illustrates the possible molecular mechanism of the AGE and the RAGE reactions in the pathogenesis of diabetic neuropathy. The AGEs exert injurious processes in the endoneurium through direct toxicity to nerve tissues together with endoneurial microangiopathy (Figure 1.7). As a result, both microangiopathic processes and neural dysfunction ensue, leading to the sensation of pain or nerve conduction delay [6].

In vitro, Schwann cells underwent apoptotic processes when exposed to a high AGE environment [67]. When the axonal cytoskeletons of tubulin and neurofilaments get glycated to stagnate axonal transport, this will result in the distal fiber degeneration [63]. Furthermore, the glycation of basement membrane collagen, laminin and fibronectin can impair the regenerative process in diabetic nerves [68, 69].

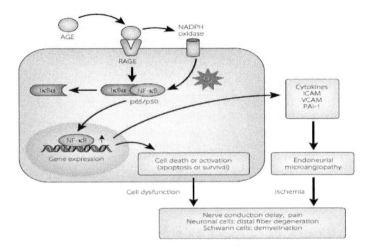

**Figure1.7: Advanced glycation end-products (AGE) and receptor for AGE (RAGE) reactions in the pathogenesis of diabetic neuropathy (Adapted from reference 6).**

Transgenic mice with enhanced expression of the RAGE in endothelial cells showed accelerated neuropathic changes in the diabetic condition, demonstrated by more severe structural changes and delayed NCV [70].

Diabetic mice lacking the RAGE gene were protective against the induction of neuropathy [71]. Thus, these findings support the highly important role of AGE in the development of diabetic neuropathy. Furthermore, there is indirect evidence which indicates the role of AGE in neuropathy. This indirect evidence is the aminoguanidine effect on experimental diabetic neuropathy [72-74]. This compound was found to inhibit the formation of AGEs, concurrently with the improvement of endoneurial blood flow[72], NCV, Na,K-ATPase activity and myelinated fiber structure[73, 74]. It is also noted that aminoguanidine effects might be mediated by its alternate action as an inducible nitric oxide synthase (iNOS) inhibitor or an anti-oxidative function [75].

In a recent study, it had been shown that animals given AGE exogenously showed significant NCV delay resembling that found in experimental diabetic neuropathy (Figure 1.8) [76]. So far still there is no proved effective compound that can suppress the AGEs formation in vivo and thus improve diabetic neuropathy in humans, however, preliminary clinical trials of anti-glycation agent, benfotiamine, showed some efficacy for diabetic neuropathy [77].

### 1.2.3 The Oxidative Stress

The generation of free radicals is known to be a major causative factor of diabetic neuropathy through accelerated glycolytic process [78, 79].

In fact, there are a lot of data which demonstrate that oxidative stress-induced tissue injury in the peripheral nerve in experimental diabetes [46, 74, 78]. Accordingly, trials have been conducted to inhibit neuropathy with antioxidants [80, 81]. Particularly, a-lipoic acid has been used for the suppression of oxidative stress in experimental diabetic rats and it was found that it improved NCV delay; nerve blood flow and nerve structure [82-84].

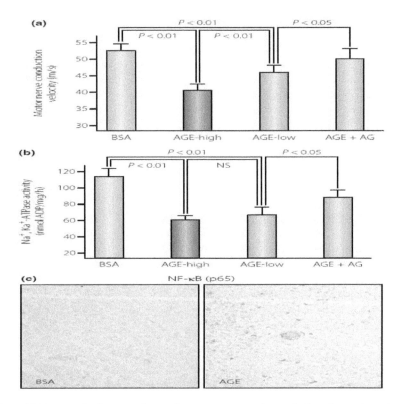

Figure1.8:Neuropathy in normal rats given exogenous advanced glycation end-products
(AGE).Rats given AGE showed (a) a significant delay of motor nerve conduction
velocity and (b) suppression of nerve Na,KATPase activity, whereas no effects were
detected in bovine serum albumin (BSA)-treated rats. Such suppression was corrected by
co-treatment with aminoguanidine (AG), an inhibitor of glycation and nitric oxide.
(c) On the sections, AGE-treated rats showed strong expression of nuclear factor-kB on
the nuclei of endothelial cells of microvessels and Schwann cells (Adapted from
reference [61]).

Both the polyol pathway and the AGEs formation produce a large amount of oxidants, and ARI

treatment can reduce the oxidative nerve injury [85, 86]. In diabetic patients, a-Lipoic acid was

found to be effective to some extent to reduce neuropathic symptoms. However, further studies

are required to confirm whether this anti- oxidant is actually effective to reduce or inhibit the

progression of the diabetic neuropathy [87].

## 1.2.4 PKC Activity

PKC is considered to be crucial in nerve function and it plays a significant role in the pathogenesis of diabetic neuropathy [88, 89]. However, the nerve tissues alterations are complicated and their supportive endoneurial vascular system, as the major enzymes of collateral glycolytic pathway are different between these two tissues [61] (Figure 1.5). Such heterogeneous tissue composition might explain the different findings on PKC activity in diabetic nerves. Nakamura et al. 1999, did not find any significant change of PKC activity in the homogenized whole peripheral nerve tissues in STZ diabetic rats, although PKC-b specific inhibitor improved NCV delay and nerve blood flow [90].In contrast, Soroku Yagihashi etal 2011 [6] reported reduced PKC activity in cultured Schwann cells exposed to high glucose [91].

Experimental studies showed potentially promising results of PKC-b-specific inhibitor on neuropathic changes in STZ-induced diabetic rats [92, 93]. Despite extensive researches, the clinical trials were not successful, partly was due to the high improvement rate in the placebo group [94]. Other PKC isoforms were also implicated in the pathological of diabetic neuropathy and inhibitors for these isoforms are being investigated [95, 96].

## 1.2.5 Pro inflammatory Processes

There is strong experimental evidence that shows nerve tissues in diabetes undergo a pro-inflammatory process which presents symptoms and accelerates the development of neuropathy [97, 98]. Figure 1.9 demonstrates the pro-inflammatory reactions in the experimental diabetic neuropathy.

The arachidonic acid pathway would be activated, resulting in increase in cyclooxygenase (COX)-2 in the peripheral nerves of STZ diabetic rats. This eventually leads to the correction of the nerve blood flow and NCV delay [99]. To confirm these data, COX-2 gene-deficient mice were shown to be protective for NCV delay after STZ-induced hyperglycemia [100]. In diabetic nerves, the pro-inflammatory condition activated the stress-kinase, mitogen-activated protein (MAP)-

kinase [101]. So, the MAP-kinase is potentially a target for a new treatment of diabetic neuropathy [102, 103].

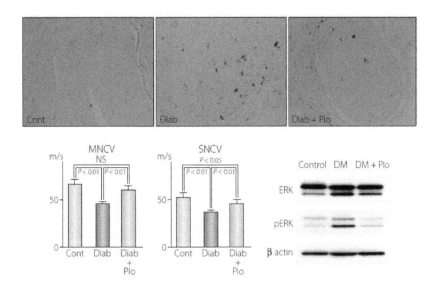

**Figure1.9: Pro-inflammatory reactions and experimental diabetic neuropathy. In the sciatic nerve of STZ-induced diabetic rats, there were many macrophages stained positive for ED1 (upper center). Migration of macrophages was inhibited when diabetic rats were treated with pioglitazone (upper right). Pioglitazone treatment also corrected the delay of motor nerve conduction velocity (MNCV) and sensory nerve conduction velocity (SNCV), and activation of extracellular signal-regulated kinase (ERK), one of mitogen activated protein kinases (MAPK)(adapted from reference 104).**

Because a pro-inflammatory reaction is induced by the polyol pathway hyperactivity or increased AGEs formation which could reflect to what extent the pro-inflammatory process is a single initiating or influential factor for the development of neuropathy. Ischemia reperfusion might also increase the inflammation to which diabetic nerves are susceptible [59, 60].With increasing data about the role of inflammation, trials to reduce or inhibit the pain symptoms or neuropathy itself are now carried out with the specific target of cytokines or cellular signals [105-107]. The insufficiency of the cellular and trophic Factors plays an important role in the pathogenesis of diabetic neuropathy [108-113]. However, due to the failed trials of nerve growth factor (NGF) application to reduce or inhibit the neuropathy [114], efforts have now been made to more efficiently deliver or produce trophic factors at the target tissues by introducing gene therapy or

cell transplantations techniques[42, 115, 116].

Furthermore, recent studies have shown a new pathological insight of the neuropathy. In

diabetic neurons, there are chimeric cells that are a combination of resident Schwann cells or

neuronal cells and migrated proinsulin-producing cells derived from bone marrow [117].

## 1.3 Treatment Directions of DPN

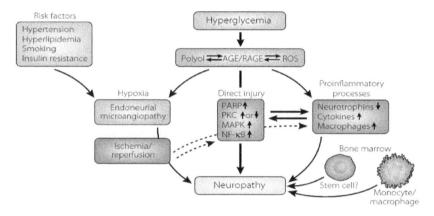

**Figure1.10: Summary of pathogenetic mechanisms of diabetic neuropathy (Adapted from reference 6).**

The chronic hyperglycemia can cause downstream metabolic cascades of polyol pathway

hyperactivity, advanced glycation end-products (AGE)/receptor for AGE (RAGE) reactions and

increased reactive oxygen species (ROS).These metabolic pathways cascades affect both

endoneurial microvessels and neural tissues and enhance the neuropathy pathogenesis process.

In addition, ischemia/reperfusion might enhance nerve injury, which is partly mediated by

inflammatory reactions [6].The following multiple Risk factors which include; insulin resistance,

hypertension, hyperlipidemia and smoking can be also important contributors to the

development of neuropathy. Based on the proposed mechanisms of neuropathy so far (Figure

1.10), researchers have been continuously trying to develop effective preparations for the

treatment of neuropathy. However, to date, there are only a few agents available in few countries; ARI (epalrestat) in Japan and a-lipoic acid (thioctic acid) in Germany. Other agents, such as benfotiamine as an anti-glycation agent, PKC-b-inhibitor (ruboxitaurine) or NGF were unfortunately unsuccessful at the final stage of RCTs.

Nevertheless, there are novel findings which emphasize the importance of diabetic neuropathy for patient care and direction of treatment in diabetes. These novel findings include;

The first novel finding is the demonstration that autonomic neuropathy in the bone marrow impaired activation and migration of endothelial precursor cells (EPC), which might determine the fate of vascular complications [118]. The second novel finding is represented by the discovery of the fact that the vagus nerve conveys signals for regeneration of islet b-cells [119]. The early inhibition of causative factors is highly important not only to stop, but also to reverse the lesions. In this setting, the combination of several inhibitors might be required. Neuropathy has long been regarded as a disorder of the most distal (peripheral) portion of the body.

Effects of hyperglycemia on the nervous system have now been shown to be a much more serious condition. Since, neuropathy itself is an important trigger for systemic abnormalities in diabetic patients, more investigatory trials on the nerve changes in the pancreas, liver and other related organs are required to improve the understanding of the whole body in diabetic patients and to develop effective treatment of this disease.

## 1.4.0 Clinical diagnosis of DPN

The DPN disease spectrum ranges from asymptomatic cases in which the neurological deficit may be discovered incidentally during a routine neurological examination, to highly debilitating ones. However, diabetic somatic neuropathies do constitute a paradox: at one extreme there are patients with severe neuropathic symptoms who on examination may have only a minimal deficit, whereas at the other extreme are those with insensate feet who are asymptomatic and may first present with foot ulcers. DPN cannot be diagnosed without a careful clinical examination and the absence of symptoms must never be taken as indication of the absence of neuropathy. The importance of excluding non-diabetic causes of neuropathy was clarified in the Rochester Diabetic Neuropathy Study, in which up to 10% of peripheral neuropathy in diabetic patients, was of non-diabetic causation [120]. DPN is by far the most common of all the diabetic neuropathies and may be divided into the following two main types: acute sensory neuropathy and chronic sensorimotor neuropathy.

Chronic sensorimotor neuropathy is by far the most common form of DPN. It is usually of insidious onset and may be present at the diagnosis of type 2 diabetes (T2DM) in up to 10% of patients. Whereas up to 50% of patients with chronic DPN may be asymptomatic, 10-20% may experience bothering symptoms sufficient to warrant specific therapy. Any patient with diabetic neuropathy should be considered to be at potential risk of foot ulceration or injury and should receive comprehensive preventive education and referral to a podiatrist as necessary. DPN late sequelae include; foot ulceration, Charcot neuroarthropathy, and occasionally amputation, which in many cases should be preventable.

Further to the results of clinical examination, the Electro-diagnostic studying is the main tool to confirm the diagnosis of DPN [121].

Electro-diagnosis in DPN usually shows sign of a distal axonopathy. On nerve conduction studies (NCS), the diagnosis of DPN requires abnormalities affecting at least two nerves, one of which must be the sural nerve [122] which is the sensory nerve in the leg calf region. NCS should include unilateral peroneal, tibial, and median motor responses, sural and median sensory responses, and tibial F-waves. Ulnar motor and sensory responses may be tested [123]. Unilateral studies are appropriate given the symmetrical nature of the condition [124]. The NCS can be used both to diagnose DPN and to identify patients with diabetes mellitus at risk for developing the DPN [125] and the Electromyography (EMG) can be used to screen for other processes such as lumbo-sacral radiculopathy. In DPN, EMG may show signs of denervation in distal muscles that can indicate motor fiber damage, even without abnormalities on NCSs [126]. It is critical to consider other syndromes if the clinical phenotype or the electrophysiological profile is indicative. It should be noted that chronic inflammatory demyelinating polyradiculoneuropathy may be missed in diabetic patients with, and these individuals can have a positive response to treatment [127].

Conventional NCSs can assess only large fiber function. However, sympathetic skin responses (SSR) can be used to assess small fiber disease, though its diagnostic performance appears to be limited in diabetic patients [128]. More frequently, small fiber neuropathy is diagnosed based on symptoms of neuropathic pain, impaired temperature/pain sensation, and autonomic dysfunction [129]. Because chronic DPN is a length-dependent process, the sensory manifestations are mainly involving the lower limbs, although, in more severe cases, the fingers and hands may also be affected. In the clinical assessment of patients, a number of simple symptom/screening questionnaires are available to record symptom quality and severity. These tools include the Michigan Neuropathy Screening Instrument, which is a brief 15-item questionnaire [130]. It is also increasingly recognized that both symptoms and deficits may have an adverse effect on quality of life in diabetic neuropathy [131].Similarly, composite scores such as a modified Neuropathy Disability Score (NDS) is increasingly used to assess clinical signs [132].

## 1.5The Therapeutic Options of DPN

In spite of multiple advances in treatment of DPN, the current medications have limited efficacy. The currently used drugs for DPN include the following;

- Antidepressants which can be further subdivided in to;

  - Tricyclic antidepressants, such as amitriptyline,

  - Other types of antidepressants, such as duloxetine and, paroxetine.

- Anticonvulsants, such as pregabalin (Lyrica), gabapentin (Gabarone, Neurontin), carbamazepine, and lamotrigine (Lamictal).

- Opioids and opioid-like drugs, such as controlled-release oxycodone and tramadol (Ultram), an opioid that also acts as an antidepressant.

- Furthermore, although some types of pain medications have been known to be effective for pain reduction in painful DPN, however, many patients with DPN are unable to achieve a level of pain relief that is greater than 30% to 50% [133], and the long-term use of these conventional medications may lead to significant serious side effects [134, 135].

In addition, different groups of drugs are either still of very restricted clinical use to specific countries or under ongoing research. These drugs include; ARIs which target the AR in the polyol pathway, anti-glycation agents and anti-oxidative agents (a Lipoic acid), are considered potentially new drugs for DPN treatment.

Some experts are not recommending the use of the currently available drugs for DPN in older adults, because of the potential seriousness of the side effects and presence of multiple co morbidities. Thus, the development of alternative new therapy to manage the diabetes complications such as the DPN remains a high priority.

## 1.6.0 DPN in Traditional Chinese Medicine (TCM)

TCM is a system of healing that originated thousands of years ago and it has evolved into a well-developed, coherent system of medicine which based on the meridian theory uses several modalities to treat and/ or prevent illness. The commonly used therapeutic methods in TCM include; acupuncture/moxibustion, Chinese herbal medicine, diet therapy, mind/body exercises (Qigong and Tai Chi), and Tui Na (Chinese massage) [136].

In TCM, the human body and its functioning are seen as a holistic structure. Based on this perspective, there is no single body part or symptom can be analyzed separately from its relation to the whole body. Unlike Western medicine, which continuously tries to discover a specific causative factor for a particular illness, TCM looks at patterns of disharmony, which include all presenting signs and symptoms as well as patients' emotional and psychological responses. Human beings are seen an integral part of nature, and according to TCM, health results from maintaining balance and harmony within the body and between the body and nature. The human body is considered as the microsome and the nature (the universe) is considered to be the macrosome [137].

TCM includes two main basic theories which explain and describe phenomena in nature, including human beings: Yin-Yang Theory and the Five Phases or Five Element Theory.

Yin and Yang are complementary and contradictory used to describe how things function in relation to each other (microsome) and to the universe (macrosome). They are interdependent which means that one cannot exist without the other, and they have the ability to transform into each other. The traditional Yin-Yang symbol (Figure 1.11) shows dark and light colored sides. The dark side represents the Yin flowing into the Yang (the light side) and vice versa. The dots within each side show that there is always a bit of Yin within Yang and a bit of Yang within Yin; which means there are no absolutes. The Yin and Yang characteristics give the basis of differentiation of all physiological functions of the body, as well as the signs and symptoms of diseases [137].

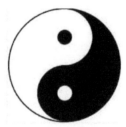

**Figure1.11: Yin and Yang Characteristics of Traditional Chinese Medicine.**

Yin and Yang are continually in dynamic state of flux and always looking for the balance point. The Yin Chinese character originally is demonstrated as the shady side of a slope. The qualitative characteristics of the Yin include; cold, stillness, darkness, inwardness, passivity, decrease, and downwardness. Furthermore, Yin would also represent the female, negative, darkness, softness, moisture, night-time, even numbers and docile aspects of things. However, the Yang Chinese character originally meant the sunny side of the slope, and the qualitative characteristics of Yang include; heat, movement, brightness, stimulation, excitement, increase, and upwardness [138]. In addition to that Yang represents the male, positive, brightness, hardness, dryness, day-time, odd numbers and dominant aspects.

The ancient scholars treated this natural phenomenon (Yin and Yang continuous flux status to achieve the balance point) as a natural universal law. Traditional Chinese Medicine views the healthy human body as an entity in yin yang equilibrium (balance) [137]. The diseases that are characterized by coldness, weakness, slowness, and under-activity are considered Yin (e.g., hypothyroidism: generalized fatigability, cold limbs, and slow metabolism). The clinical disorders that manifest as strength, jerky (forceful) movement, heat, and over activity are Yang (e.g., acute infections with high temperature and excessive perspiration).

The second TCM theory is the theory of five elements, in Chinese it is called *Wu Xing*, is a way of classifying phenomena in terms of five basic processes represented by the elements which include; wood, fire, earth, metal, and water. According to TCM, a dynamic balance and relationship among these five elements do exist. If this balance is disturbed, pathological changes can occur. The clockwise movement of one element into the next (wood, fire, earth, and so forth) whereby one element generates, acts on, or promotes the following element, is referred to as the Sheng cycle. The Ke cycle (Figure 1.12) represents an element acting on or controlling another element in a different order [136, 137].

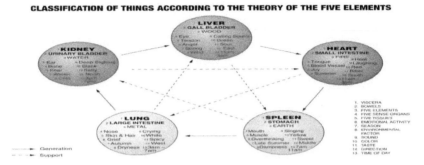

**Figure1.12: Five Elements theory of Traditional Chinese Medicine.**

Within this model of five elements, each element is associated with an organ. For example, Wood is associated with the liver, fire with the heart, earth with the spleen-pancreas-stomach, metal with the lungs, and water with the kidneys. Furthermore, other phenomena, such as seasons, cardinal directions, weather, emotions, and, color are also associated with each element. Within the TCM model, diagnostic information is gained by finding out patients' predominant emotion(s), favorite season, and color [137].

Within five element theory, there are four main relationships or ways in which the elements interact. These relationships can be distributed between two categories as following (Table1. 2);

**Table 1.2: The relationships of the five elements in TCM**

| Normal Category | Abnormal Category |
| --- | --- |
| 1. **Inter generating** (Xiang-Shang) which generating and promoting each other like the relationship of the mother and child | 1. **Over-Restricting (Over Controlling)** (Xiang-Cheng) |
| 2. **Inter restricting** (Xiang Ke) | 2. **Reverse Restraining** (Xiang Wu) |

## 1.6.1 Key Concepts within TCM

The key concepts within TCM are the following;
- Qi
- Meridians
- Jing (Essence)
- Shen (Spirit)
- Blood
- Fluids

## 1.6.1.1 Qi

The Qi (pronounced "chi") in English and it might mean the vital energy. It is recognized in terms of function rather than as a substance, and it is what allows us to be active and maintain all life functions. The origins of Qi include; prenatal (congenital) Qi, which is inherited from our parents—and postnatal (acquired) Qi, which is extracted from air and food [138].

There are two major patterns of disharmony are associated with Qi. The deficient Qi which appears when there is insufficient Qi to conduct the life functions. Deficient Qi may impact one or more organs or the entire body, in which case the patient may complain of; lethargy, fatigue, and lack of desire to move. Stagnant Qi is defined as the impairment of the normal movement of Qi through the meridians which may manifest as pains in the body [138].

## 1.6.1.2 The Meridians

Meridians are the pathways through which Qi is normally flowing throughout the body. There are 12 regular meridians and 8 extra meridians. The 12 main meridians correspond to 12 major functions (organs) of the body (such as spleen, liver, kidney, heart). The TCM concept of organs corresponds very slightly to the Western medicine (WM) concept. While, WM view is restricted primarily to function, TCM associates specific functions, tastes, emotions, colors, and symptoms, with each organ. Qi should flow in the correct quantity and quality through the meridians and organs for health to be maintained. Acupuncture, the insertion of thin, solid metal needles, is performed on 1 or more of the 361 acupuncture points distributed along these various meridians in order to regulate and promote the proper flow of Qi [139]. Other techniques may be used to stimulate acupuncture points, such as moxibustion, in which the herb moxa (Artemesia vulgaris) is used to warm the acupuncture point either above (Indirect Moxibustion) or on the skin (Direct Moxibustion) [137].

### 1.6.1.3 The Jing

Jing can be translated as essence, and is defined as the blueprint substance of all organic life. Qi is responsible for the ongoing day-to-day movements and function of the body, whereas Jing can be considered an individual's constitutional blueprints. Jing is stored in the kidneys [138].

### 1.6.1.4 Shen

Shen can be defined as the spirit of the individual. Shen is the vitality behind Jing and Qi in the human body. The three elements together—Qi, Jing, and Shen—are referred to collectively in TCM as the "Three Treasures" and are believed to be the main essential components of human life [139].

### 1.6.1.5 Blood

In TCM, the main blood function is to circulate through the body, nourishing and moistening the various organs and tissues. Blood disharmonies may manifest as "deficient" blood or congealed (stagnant or coagulated) blood. The deficient blood affects the entire body and it may manifest as a dull complexion, dry skin, and dizziness. However, congealed blood may present as sharp, stabbing pains which generally will be accompanied by tumors, cysts, or swelling of the organs (i.e., the liver) [138]. In TCM, the key organs associated with blood are the spleen, liver, and heart.

### 1.6.1.6 Fluids

Fluids are bodily liquids other than blood and include saliva, sweat, urine, tears, and semen. Fluids function is to moisten both the exterior (skin and hair) and the internal organs. Disharmonies of fluids may result in dryness and excess heat. The key organs involved in the formation, distribution, and excretion of fluids are the kidneys, spleen, and lungs [140].

### 1.6.2 Diagnosis in TCM

When assessing patients with a chronic illness such as diabetes, TCM practitioners take a detailed, multi-system case history and supplement this information with observations that give information about the state of the patient's health. These observations include the tongue shape, color, and coating; the expression and color of the face; the odor of the breath and body; and the strength, rhythm, and quality of the pulse. The TCM practitioners will also palpate along meridians to assess the tenderness and sensitivity of the points that may indicate a blockage in the flow of Qi at those tender points [141].

One of the most common ways of differentiating symptoms and syndromes in TCM is according to the Eight Principles which include the following—four pairs of polar opposites: Yin and Yang, Interior and Exterior, Cold and Heat, and Deficiency and Excess [137].

### 1.6.3 TCM Classification of Diabetes

The Chinese language uses two terms for diabetes. The traditional name, Xiao-ke, correlates closely with diabetes. Xiao-ke syndrome means wasting and thirsting. The more modern term, Tang-niao-bing, means sugar urine illness. Reference to diabetes by the traditional term appears in the earliest texts, including the first medical text in Chinese history; *The Yellow Emperor's Inner Classic (Huang Di Nei Jing)* [137].

According to TCM, Diabetes is classically divided into three types: upper, middle, and lower Xiao-ke. Each type has its characteristic symptoms.

The upper Xiao-ke type is closely associated with the lungs and is characterized by excessive thirst, the middle Xiao-ke type is closely associated with stomach and is characterized by excessive hunger, and the lower Xiao-ke type is closely associated with kidney and is characterized by excessive urination. All the three types are associated with Yin deficiency. At some point during the course of the disease, most people with diabetes manifest mixed symptoms of all three types.

According to TCM, Xiao-ke is attributed to three main factors:

➢    Improper diet

➢    Emotional disturbances (stress, anxiety, depression,) and

➢    A constitutional Yin deficiency (fatigue, weakness, lethargy, pale complexion) [142].

TCM diagnoses may sound esoteric. In the case of a person with diabetes presenting with symptoms of excessive thirst, the TCM diagnosis can be described as kidney Yin deficiency along with lung Yin deficiency and internal heat that consumes fluids, thus bringing on wasting and thirsting [142].

In TCM and based on the Syndrome Differentiation approach, DPN is believed to be rooted from qi-yin deficiency and presented with blood stasis and collateral obstruction. Multiple organs are affected which include the liver, kidney, spleen and stomach in particular [137].

According to TCM, the DPN is pertaining to the category of flaccidity syndrome and Bi-obstruction syndrome. Clinically, DPN is characterized by sensory disturbances in form of a symmetrical numbness, pain, burning sensation and dyskinesia in the distal limbs, especially the lower limbs, and in severe cases, even by ulceration, necrosis and amputation, which is the major cause of disability of diabetes mellitus and severely affects the diabetic patients quality of life; physically and mentally [137].

## 1.6.4 Pathogenesis of DPN according to TCM

### 1. Qi-yin deficiency is the root aspect of DPN and blood-stasis and collateral obstruction are its' manifestation

Although in TCM, diabetes mellitus is called Xiao Ke, however its complications of peripheral neuropathy are not found in the ancient Chinese medical books. The DPN symptoms such as limb numbness, pain and burning are seen in Flaccidity Syndrome and Bi-obstruction Syndrome. In TCM, DPN is believed to be caused by qi-yin deficiency and even yin deficiency affecting yang and subsequently yin-yang insufficiency in chronic diabetes mellitus. Qi-yin insufficiency fails to nourish meridians, collaterals and skin, and the yang-qi cannot reach the distal limbs, manifesting as limb numbness and weakness, skin coldness or dryness [137].

In TCM theory, chronic disorders always can lead to deficiency and blood-stasis and affect collaterals and are difficult to treat and cure. Insufficient yang-qi cannot move blood and deficient yin-fluid cannot nourish meridians and collaterals, causing meridian-collateral

28

obstruction [137]. In addition to that, insufficiency of healthy qi, phlegm turbidity, cold pathogens or damp-heat may further obstruct meridians and collaterals and cause qi-blood stagnation. Meridian-collateral blockage gives rise to aches and various types of sensation in the distal limbs. Many research results have demonstrated that, in DPN patients, slowing blood flow and increasing platelet aggregation and whole blood viscosity affect the endothelium cells of small vessels, activate the functions of endothelium cells, slow down blood flow, and induce basement membrane degeneration and glass transition, and finally cause obstruction of small blood vessels[137]. In WM, the microangiopathies and hemodynamics changes are considered as the major causative factors of DPN pathogenesis. HUANG You-min [137] believed that hemodynamics change, microcirculation disturbance, endothelium cell impairment, high blood viscosity, altered vascular shape and chemical components of diabetic vascular diseases are similar to the condition of blood-stasis syndrome in TCM. DPN can be differentiated into several syndromes, but blood-stasis stays throughout the whole process and becomes the primary pathogenic factor.

**2. In focus liver, kidney, spleen and stomach are involved**

DPN is a complicated illness. In the early stage, the lung and stomach are involved, but later the liver and kidney are affected. The spleen functions to process food and drink and becomes the source of qi and blood; the stomach contains more qi and blood and is named as the sea of food and drink. The spleen and stomach are together called postnatal foundation. However, Kidneys house essence and have yuan primordial yin and yuan primordial yang, and are considered as the prenatal foundation. The spleen and kidney depend on each other and spleen-kidney insufficiency plays a significant role in the development of DPN. Deficiency of kidney and spleen, yin and yang hypofunction and qi-blood insufficiency will result in malnourishment of meridians and collaterals; in the long run, the liver and kidney are affected to generate wind, which eventually enters the collaterals to result in limb pain and dyskinesia. In clinical practice, the affected organs should be differentiated at first to make correct diagnosis and treatment [137].

### 1.6.5 TCM Therapies

TCM management methodology is not concerned with measuring and monitoring blood glucose levels in diabetic patients. However, treatment is individualized and tailored toward assessing and treating the symptoms that compose patterns of deficiency and disharmony.

Acupuncture and moxibustion traditionally have been used in the treatment of diabetes to reduce blood glucose levels. The clinical and experimental studies have demonstrated that acupuncture treatment has a beneficial effect on lowering serum glucose levels [137].

A typical acupuncture treatment involves needling 4–12 points and the needles will be kept in place for ~10–30 min. Needles may be stimulated manually or by using a small electrical current. In addition, the TCM practitioner may warm the points with moxibustion including warm needling.

DPN as one of the most common complications of T2DM, it occurs most often in the distal extremities and typically affects the sensory, motor, and autonomic systems. Acupuncture treatment has been demonstrated a potentially beneficial effect particularly on neuropathic pain. The effects of acupuncture, specifically on pain, might be mediated in part by the release of endogenous opioids from the spinal cord, brainstem, and hypothalamus. In addition, it has been demonstrated that neurotransmitters, such as serotonin and substance P, are released during acupuncture treatments. Furthermore, increases in local blood flow, vasodilatation and increased levels of cortisol have also been demonstrated with acupuncture treatment [139]. Up to 300% rise in plethysmographic recordings of blood flow has been reported in the digits of limbs stimulated with electro-acupuncture treatment [139].

Since the pathogenesis of DPN is still uncertain, there is no cure for it so far. However, in recent years, acupuncture treatment has been increasingly used to treat DPN and promising results have been achieved [137].

## 1.6.6 Treatment Principles of DPN according to TCM Theory

### 1. Concentrating on the root and the branch aspects to unblock

Based on above TCM analysis of the DPN pathogenesis, acupuncture treatment should concentrate on enriching qi and yin or warming yang. Blood-stasis is the major pathological factor and the acupuncture treatment should thus focus on unblocking therapy for blood activation and blood-stasis removal. Moxibustion can be used also to enrich qi and warm yang for unblocking therapy [137].

### 2. Concentrating on the whole body to regulate zang-fu organs

The meridian and collateral carry qi and blood, which are transformed by zang-fu organs; therefore, zang-fu organs are the base of meridians' function. Although the clinical symptoms of DPN are located in the limbs, but they are caused by the dysfunction of the liver, kidney, spleen and stomach; therefore, the acupuncture treatment, in addition to limbs acupoints, should wholly focus on regulating the zang-fu organs, to produce qi and blood as well as balance yin and yang. Acupoints are chosen according of acupuncture theory, and some specific acupoints such as Yuan-primary points, He-Sea points and Luo-Connecting points of liver, kidney, spleen and stomach meridians as well as the back-Shu or front-Mu points of associated zang-fu organs are often selected. Acupuncture treatment is performed to balance zang-fu organs, harmonize yin and yang to make a whole regulation and balance to the human body [137].

It is very important to note that because of poor peripheral circulation in patients with DPN and slowed healing of skin infections and ulcerations, acupuncture needling of the lower extremities in such patients should be performed with extreme caution and sterile technique. However, generally, acupuncture treatment seems to be a relatively safe form of treatment. An extensive international literature search depicted only 193 adverse events (including relatively minor events, such as bruising and dizziness) over time period of 15-years. There have been also about 86 reported cases of hepatitis B and 1 case of HIV transmission. However, it should be well noted that in all of these cases, non-disposable needles were used [137].

Acupuncture is one of the oldest and most commonly used forms of alternative medicine, has existed for more than 2500 years. Acupuncture is a meridian-based therapy. In traditional acupuncture, needles are inserted into precisely defined, specific points on the body, each of which has distinct therapeutic actions [140]. Acupuncture has long been used in East Asia for pain relief based on the Qi theory, and acupuncture can reduce pain (acupuncture analgesia) by regulating the imbalance of Qi. In the WM, acupuncture has increasingly been a recent subject of research in the treatment of chronic pain. Acupuncture analgesia might be explained by the following scientific mechanisms: local effect [141], segmental analgesia [140] extra-segmental analgesia [140] and central regulation of the limbic system [142, 143]. In a recent, well-designed meta-analysis of randomized clinical trials (RCTs) with data from 17,922 patients, it was reported that acupuncture is more effective for treating chronic pain than both; sham acupuncture and no treatment [144, 145]. With increasing basic and clinical evidence, acupuncture is being more widely used for various types of pain control, including the pain of neuropathy.

## 1.6.7 Acupuncture Analgesia

Acupuncture Analgesia (AA) can be defined as analgesia produced by insertion of acupuncture needles at certain acupuncture points in the body. These will activate the small myelinated nerve fibers in the muscles which in turn will transmit the neural signals to the spinal cord and will activate the following three neural centers; the spinal cord, midbrain and pituitary hypothalamus to produce analgesia.

The mechanism of AA has been studied extensively since 1965 and it is a main branch in Experimental Acupuncture Science. The General rules in acupuncture analgesia are the following:

➢ Acupuncture is potentially able to relief acute and chronic pains.

> ➤ Acupuncture can relief superficial, deep, visceral and referred pains.

> ➤ The optimal analgesia effects occur at time of 20-40 min during manipulation.

> ➤ The analgesia effect depends on constant manipulation. Once the manipulation stops, the analgesia effect gradually decline. The half-value period is 16 min.

The action of AA involves both; local mechanism and Systemic mechanism (Neuro-humoral mechanism); however, these AA mechanisms can be further subdivided and explained by the following scientific mechanisms:

> ➤ The local effect which is mediated by adenosine A1 receptors [146, 147],

> ➤ The segmental analgesia, which based on the pain gate control theory [148]

> ➤ The extra-segmental analgesia, which demonstrates the releasing of opioid peptides or descending inhibitory pain control [149, 150] and

> ➤ The central regulation of the limbic system, which is relevant to the affective component of pain [151].

So, at the first stage; Needle insertion will activate Mast cells and nerve endings (Figure 1.13 & Figure 1.14). These nerve endings express various mechanic-sensitive receptors which can sense many types of mechanical stimuli, stroke, touch, pressure or noxious and include both; nociceptors (pain receptors) and non-nociceptors (touch pressure receptors).

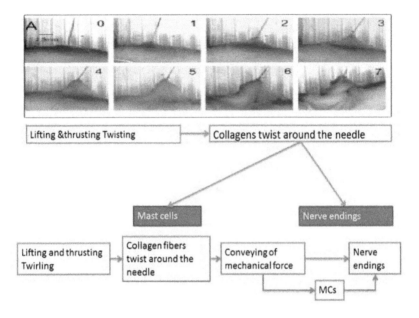

Figure1.13: The deformation of connective tissue during unidirectional twisting of acupuncture needle (adapted from the course lecture).

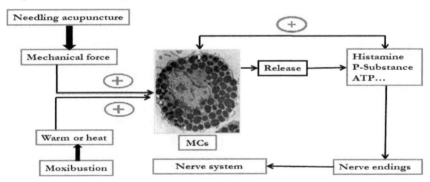

Figure1.14: Local acupoint mechanism (MCs=Mast cells) (adapted from the course lecture).

Acupuncture treatment involves multi- neurotransmitters and neuromodulators that contribute to AA which include the following;

> Endogenous opioid peptide system which include; β-Endorphin, Enkephalin and dynorphin (Figure 1.15)

➤ Classical neurotransmitters which include; 5-HT (5-Hydroxytryptamine), Acetylcholine

(Ach) and Noradrenaline

It should be noted that the manual acupuncture (MA) and electro acupuncture (EA) are widely

used nowadays and the used frequency in EA is known to be a key parameter and the effects of

EA will vary accordingly (Figure 1.15). It is generally recognized that low frequency stimulation

(LF) < 10Hz releases opioid peptides, such as beta-endorphin and enkephalin, and has a

relatively longer-lasting and generalized effect, while high frequency stimulation (HF) around 80

to 200 Hz releases different opioid peptides, such as dynorphin, and has a relatively short-term

and predominantly segmental effect [151]. In practice, it is recommended that both LF and HF be

used together as a dense-disperse (DD) wave because the DD mode can prevent nerve

accommodation and release various neurotransmitters [149, 151].

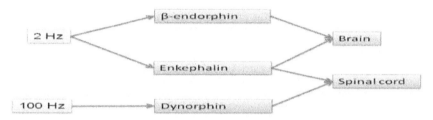

**Figure1.15: Endogenous opioid peptide system in acupuncture analgesia (Adapted from the course lecture).**

On acupuncture treatment, the nerve fibers sense the noxious stimuli and then transmit the

signals to the dorsal horn of the spinal cord and continuously ascend up to brain (Figure1.16)

which gives a rough pathway of pain perception. Although many theories have been proposed,

however, so far the exact mechanism of pain perception is still unclear.

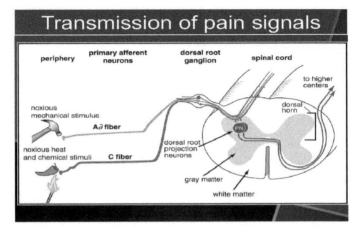

**Figure1.16: The rough pathway of pain perception (Adapted from the course lecture).**

Nevertheless, among the proposed theories of pain signals transmission is the Gate Control theory which was proposed in 1965 by Ronald Melzack & Patrick Wall, and so far, it is considered to be the most influential theory. Furthermore, another important scientific theory relevant to AA is the Diffuse Noxious Inhibitory Controls (DNIC) theory.

### 1.6.7.1 The Gate Control Theory

This theory has explained why pain sensation can be quickly relieved by moderate mechanical stimulus. Gate Control machinery focuses on the spinal cord (Figure1.17).

The Control Gate decides the noxious signal transmit to brain or not. The afferent nerves of this gate include; the projection neurons which receive the signal from the nerve fibers and transmit it to the brain as well as the SG cells which are inter-neurons (Figure1.18).

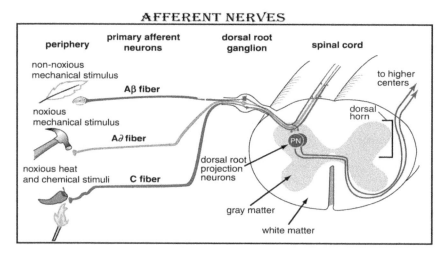

Figure1.17:The Gate Control Theory (Adapted from the course lecture).

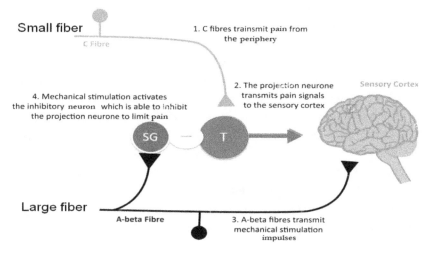

Figure1.18: The Gate Control mechanism of pain perception in Acupuncture Analgesia (Adapted from the course lecture).

The input signal pathways to the control gate include two pathways;

1. Small nerve fibers (C-fibers) pain pathway

2. Large fibers (A-beta fibers) sensory neural pathway

Both pathways are connected to projection cells (T cells) which carry signals through the spino-thalamic tract. In normal situations the Gate is closed, however, when C fibers are activated by noxious stimuli and input signals to the projection cells (T cell) will open the Gate and pain signal will be transmitted and perceived. In the contrary when the large fibers (A-beta fibers) are activated, the inhibitory neurons (SG) get activated and the projection cells are also activated and the transmission of pain signals through them is prevented by the inhibitory neurons and the Gate remains closed, so no pain perception occurs as the brain does not receive the signal.

The outcome of the basic research indicates that the acupuncture can activate both; the large nerve fibers (Aα, Aβ, Aδ) and the small nerve fibers (C fibers). Although, the gate theory involves the large nerve fibers (Aα, Aβ and Aδ fibers), however, the C fibers are mainly involved in systemic mechanism. So accordingly, the Gate Control theory explains why moderate acupuncture manipulation can relieve pain and it shows that the stronger manipulations are applied, the better the analgesic effect occur. However, systemic mechanism might give the explanation for the acupuncture analgesic effects through the activation of C fibers by stronger stimulation.

### 1.6.7.2 The Diffuse Noxious Inhibitory Controls (DNIC)

The phenomenon of pain inhibiting pain has been known empirically for centuries. This phenomenon reveals diffuse inhibitory mechanisms which can be activated by a painful focus. Noxious stimuli activate a surround inhibition that sharpens contrast between the stimulus zone and adjacent areas. This sharpened contrast has a net enhancing effect on the perceived intensity of the painful stimulus and an analgesic effect outside the stimulated zone, so, the inhibition within the spinal cord by noxious stimulation applied to one part of the body inhibits nociception in another part of the body (Figure 1.19). This surround analgesia may explain counter irritation and acupuncture analgesia. Therefore, the acupuncture signals integrate with pain signals in brain stem, thalamus and cerebral cortex (Figure 1.19).

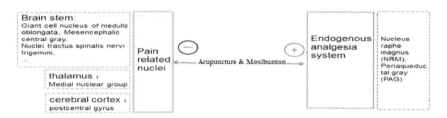

**Figure1.19: Integration of acupuncture signals with CNS (Adapted from the course lecture).**

### 1.6.7.3 The Acupuncture Tolerance and the Acupuncture Non-Responders

The AA efficiency reduces because of long-term or repeatable treatment of acupuncture. This phenomenon is called tolerance and might be mediated through cholecystokinin-octopeptide (CCK-8) in acupuncture analgesia (Figure 1.20).

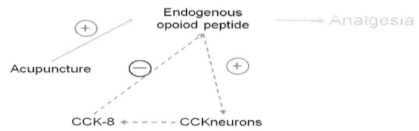

**Figure1.20: The role of Cholecystokinin-Octopeptide [CCK-8] in Acupuncture Tolerance (Adapted from the course lecture).**

Furthermore, the phenomenon of the acupuncture treatment failure (acupuncture non-responder) was written in the oldest Chinese archives of acupuncture textbooks [148]. It is stated that one in seven subjects will respond either poorly or not at all, to acupuncture treatment, and the TCM practitioners in such situations, are advised not to go further in acupuncture treatment in order to avoid causing harm to the patients [148]. Recent data from animal experiments have demonstrated the potential biochemical basis for this failure of acupuncture treatment [148] which indicates that Cholecystokinin octapeptide (CCK-8) is a powerful endogenous neuropeptide acting on the CCKA/CCKB receptors with anti-opioid activity [149,150]. The CCK-8 which is distributed in the spinal cord and the brain has been shown to have an antagonistic effect on EA analgesia [150, 151] that in turn can be reversed by CCKB receptor antagonist [149,152]. Furthermore,

Huang et al [151] has shown the reduction in the effects of EA analgesia with an intra-thecal injection of CCK-8, whereas CCKB receptor antagonist has potentiated the analgesia. So, the production of CCK-8 antagonists might be potentially implicated as a determinant of the trait of weak or non-response to acupuncture Treatment [153] Nevertheless, to date there has been no RCT of endogenous CCK levels or CCK receptor phenotyping among poor or non-responders to acupuncture compared with responders [148].

So, the main aim of this literature review study is to; make a basic analysis of the effectiveness and safety of using the acupuncture techniques in the treatment of DPN as add on complementary treatment. The analysis in this study will include a comparison between real acupuncture and other control groups which include among the others; Sham Acupuncture (SA) and usual care (without implementing any type of acupuncture). Furthermore, this study will include the conductance of the evaluation of the feasibility of implementing the acupuncture therapy as a complementary medical technique for the treatment of the DPN in a large-scale prospective clinical randomized controlled trial.

# CHAPTER 2

# MATERIALS AND METHODS

## 2.0 Materials and Methods

In this chapter, the aims and objectives of this Literature review will be defined. The process by which this literature search was conducted will be described as well as the tools of the literature search and of the quality assessment will be provided.

### 2.1 The Scope of This Research

The scope of this Literature review research is to assess the usefulness of using acupuncture as additional (add-on) or complementary treatment tool in the management of Diabetic Peripheral Neuropathy (DPN).

### 2.2 The Aim of This Research

The aim of this Literature review research is to explore the degree of effectiveness and safety of acupuncture in treating DPN.

### 2.3 The Objectives of This Research

➢ To identify the various acupuncture points (acupoints) reportedly used for treating various symptoms of DPN,

➢ To learn whether acupuncture can only improves the symptoms of DPN or whether it might have a curing potential effect by promoting the nerve regeneration which can be assessed by nerve conduction studies.

➢ To learn about the effectiveness of acupuncture in managing DPN,

➢ To identify whether there are any known side effects of acupuncture during the procedure of management of DPN,

➢ To learn whether acupuncture reduces the need for further drugs which are currently in use to alleviate the symptoms of DPN, such as opiods Or Lyrica, etc.

➢ To explore the possible influences of acupuncture on the management process of DPN.

> To collect the relevant data that would be required in a future well designed study for investigating the efficacy of acupuncture in DPN through a prospective research clinical trial which will comply with all related international guidelines and ensure robustness.

## 2.4.0 Literature Search

### 2.4.1 Literature Collecting Methods

#### 2.4.1.1 Database

An extensive systemic full text literature search of Randomized Controlled Trials [RCTs] with acupuncture treatment of DPN was conducted to evaluate the proportion of positive conclusions in the different controls in RCTs. The search strategy was defined as below. The search was carried out by making use of multiple online search engines and databases including; the Hydi academic search engine of the library of the University of Malta. This engine incorporates multiple international academic databases which are: Academic Search Complete (EBSCO), Cumulative Index to Nursing and Allied Health Literature (CINHAL) Plus with Full Text, Google Scholar, Science Direct, Wiley Online Library, Scopus, PubMed, the Medline, AMED, Cochrane libraries, EMBASE and clintrials.gov databases. Furthermore, manual searches were also carried out at the University of Malta main library as well as the Faculty of Health Sciences library.

#### 2.4.1.2 Search Strategy

English has been limited as the searching language.

The following English key words were used in order to carry out the literature search: 'acupuncture' or 'acupoints' or 'acupuncture points' or 'electro-acupuncture' or 'manual acupuncture,' "meridian", "needle, "sham acupuncture", "AND 'Peripheral Diabetic Neuropathy' or 'Diabetic Neuropathy' or 'DPN management' AND 'patients' experiences' or 'patients satisfaction'. Studies were limited to RCTs and journals in Science Citation Index (SCI).

### 2.4.1.3 Selection Criteria

### 2.4.1.3.1 Inclusion Criteria

The studies included in this meta-analysis: (1) were RCTs; (2) used needling acupuncture [Chinese Traditional manual acupuncture (MA) or/and electro-acupuncture (EA)] as the major intervention. It also included; the head and the scalp acupuncture as the secondary intervention as well as the wrist and ankle acupuncture as a comparator); and (4) were published during the past 11 years (from 2006 to 2017).

### 2.4.1.3.2 Exclusion Criteria

Studies excluded from the analysis were those considered: (1) of poor quality design (unclear randomization method, incorrect concealment, and individual assessment), (2) involved the use of Chinese herbal medicine as active treatment and (3) used active treatment of any acupuncture modalities (e.g., active acupuncture, auricular acupuncture, etc.) as control(s).

By applying the literature inclusion/exclusion criteria defined above, all complied RCTs that used acupuncture treatment for DPN, were selected. Among the selected studies, the intervention groups were treated mainly with acupuncture therapy or with some other standard therapies accompanied by acupuncture, such as Moxibustion, taking oral hypoglycemic agents, having diabetic diet and so on.

Furthermore, the parallel randomized controlled trials (RCTs) that evaluated manual or electro-acupuncture for the treatment of DPN; were also included, regardless of the language used in the publication whether it was English or Chinese.

The definition of DPN used in the reported studies conformed to the following diagnostic criteria: the patient has diabetes mellitus by internationally recognized criteria, such as the world health organization (WHO) criteria [154]; and the patient had predominantly distal symmetrical sensorimotor polyneuropathy of the limbs - other causes of sensorimotor polyneuropathy have been excluded.

Manual acupuncture was defined as manual stimulation of acupuncture points, with penetration of the skin by thin metal needles. Scalp acupuncture, acupoint injection, electro-acupuncture, moxibustion and the combination of manual acupuncture with any of the above were included in the analysis as well. However, studies involving laser acupuncture and Chinese herbal medicine trials were excluded. Eligible control groups were one of the following:

➢ Another (potentially) active treatment (Medication group),

➢ Sham acupuncture, or

➢ Usual care control group.

The RCTs that compared acupuncture plus another (potentially) active treatment versus that other (potentially) active treatment alone were also included.

## 2.4.1.4 Screening

The retrieved studies were seen and any duplicates were removed. The abstracts of the studies were screened, followed by full-text screening according to the above selection criteria. The screening was performed; with any queries being comprehensively discussed. Information on the type of controls and acupuncture efficacy conclusion from eligible studies were extracted according to the definition of outcomes.

The RCTs assessing acupuncture's efficacy for the treatment of the DPN were therefore reviewed. The parallel RCTs focused on acupuncture's efficacy were reviewed and screened for eligibility. The Scale for Assessing Scientific Quality of Investigations in Complementary and Alternative Medicine (STRICTA) [155] was modified by integrating the Jadad scale [156] with it – here subsequently termed STRICTA PLUS Scoring Scale (STRICTA-P) which is a novel tool. This newly modified STRICTA-P was used to assess RCT quality. The RCTs with STRICTA-P's score of >9 and active control treatments such as sham acupuncture or medical therapy were included in the final analysis.

The studies included in this review (Table: 2.1) were written either in the English language or

translated from Chinese into the English language using online translating tool. The included

trials were mainly carried out in China and few others in the United Kingdom (UK), or the USA.

This could be considered as a limitation, since a lot of studies on acupuncture were written in the

Chinese language or other languages like Tibetan language where online translation was not

possible. I have tried further to identify studies carried out in the Maltese environment, however;

I did not find any local Maltese study which was carried out on acupuncture use for treatment of

the Peripheral Diabetic Neuropathy in Malta so far and this literature review research is

considered to be the first of this type in the University of Malta about this subject.

**Table2.1 List of studies included in this Literature review research.*RCT stands for Random Controlled Trial.**

| No | Authors | Year | Study Design | Country |
|----|---------|------|--------------|---------|
| 1 | ZHAO Hui-ling , GAO Xin , GAO Yan-bin , et al. [157] | 2007 | RCT* | China |
| 2 | Garrow AP., et al [158] | 2014 | RCT* | UK |
| 3 | Lu M., et al. [159] | 2016 | RCT* | China |
| 4 | Jin Z., et al [160] | 2011 | RCT* | China |
| 5 | Ji XQ., et al [161] | 2010 | RCT* | China |
| 6 | Tong Y, Guo H, Han B. [162] | 2010 | RCT* | China |
| 7 | Zhang C, Ma YX, Yan Y. [163] | 2010 | RCT* | China |
| 8 | Chen YL., et al [164] | 2009 | RCT* | China |
| 9 | Jiang H, et al. [165] | 2006 | RCT* | China |
| 10 | Anne Bailey., et al [166] | 2017 | RCT* | USA |
| 11 | SUN Yuan-zheng, XU Ying-ying. [167] | 2010 | RCT* | China |
| 12 | Wang Hui, et al [168] | 2015 | RCT* | China |
| 13 | Zhao Zhixuan, et al. [169] | 2010 | RCT* | China |
| 14 | FEI Ai-hua, et al [170] | 2011 | RCT* | China |
| 15 | GAO Yu [171] | 2016 | RCT* | China |
| 16 | ZUO Lin, ZHANG Lin [172] | 2010 | RCT* | China |

## 2.5 Types of Studies

A total of 63 potentially relevant articles were retrieved during this literature search. Of these, 47

studies were excluded from this literature review because they did not meet the predetermined

selection criteria. Finally, sixteen RCTs which met the inclusion criteria and provided exclusive information about the use of acupuncture therapy for the treatment of the DPN were chosen

and were included in this literature review (Table.2.1), all are (Figure: 2.1).

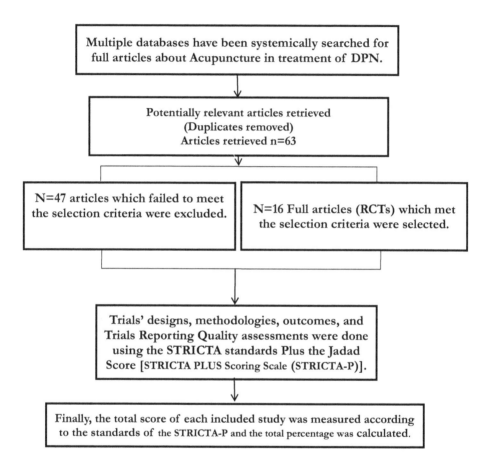

Figure2.1  Flow chart of Search

## 2.5.1 Participants

The analysed studies all together had included a total of 1037 participants.

## 2.5.2 Diagnostic Criteria

Variable diagnostic criteria for Diabetes and DPN have been implemented in the analyzed RCTs and quarter of the selected studies failed to refer to any diagnostic criteria.

**The Diabetes Diagnostic criteria used in the selected studies are the following:**

> ➢ The WHO 1999 diagnostic criteria [154].
> ➢ The American Diabetes Association (ADA) 1997 diagnostic criteria [173].
> ➢ The Chinese Medical Association, Diabetes Branch criteria.
> ➢ Adoption of the western criteria with reference to Shen Zhao yuan editor of the diabetes Chronic complications [174] and Jiang Yu-ping editor of clinical neurological disease [175].

**The DPN Diagnostic criteria used in the selected RCTs are the following:**

> ➢ The WHOPNTF on DPN diagnostic criteria
> ➢ The Chinese Medicine diagnostic criteria with reference to the Diagnostic Criteria drawn by Qian Zhaoren [176] in which TCM differentiation was done in accordance with the criteria set by Lin Lan [177].
> ➢ The Japanese simple diagnostic criteria of DPN which was revised on 2002[178].
> ➢ However, the majority had given the description of the symptoms and the signs of DPN without specifying any diagnostic criteria.

## 2.5.2 Types in Interventions

Of these 16 studies, 12 studies tested the manual acupuncture; three used both the manual and the electro-acupuncture and one study tested the warm acupuncture (warm needling).

## 2.6 Outcomes

The outcomes of the included RCTs were highly variable; however, they included various tools which generally included one of the following;

- The score of peripheral neuropathy of diabetes mellitus,
- The change of nerve conduction: velocity and
- Clinical efficacy before and after treatment in the two groups were observed.

Since most of the selected studies were done in China, they have used evaluation indexes of symptoms and signs in accordance with the Guiding Principles for Clinical Study of New Chinese Medicines [176, 177].These were graded as following;

> ➢ Marked effectiveness: The patient tells that the symptoms and signs have disappeared.
> ➢ Effectiveness: The patient tells that the symptoms and signs are reduced.
> ➢ Failure: The patient complains of no change in symptomatology.

Total efficiency rate was calculated separately and compared between treatment and control groups using the following formula;

$$Total\ efficiency(\%) = \left[\frac{Significant\ number\ of\ cases + Valid\ cases}{Total\ case\ Number}\right] X100$$

However, other included RCTs had used one of the following outcomes assessment tools;

➢ The Neuropathy Total Symptom Scale (NTSS-6),
➢ the Neuropathy Disability Score (NDS),
➢ the determination of nerve conduction velocity both sensory nerve conduction velocity (SNCV)and motor nerve conduction velocity (MNCV).

One study which was conducted in the UK (Garrow AP, et al 2014) [158] had used the following tools to assess the outcomes;

➢ The Leeds Assessment of Neuropathic Symptoms and Signs (LANSS) scale, lower limb pain (Visual Analogue Scale, VAS);
➢ Sleep Problem Scale (SPS);
➢ Measure Yourself Medical Outcome Profile (MYMOP);
➢ 36-item Short Form 36 Health Survey and
➢ Resting blood pressure (BP).

The primary outcome was the global symptom improvement measured either by a visual analogue scale (VAS) [179], or the total symptom score [180]. Where this outcome was not available, the global symptom improvement measured by whatever criteria that were determined by the authors as the primary outcome. The secondary outcomes were; the change in nerve conduction velocity measured by validated methods, the quality of life, and the adverse events.

## 2.6.1 Types of the Acupuncture Controls

The   acupuncture controls were classified into several types according to the purpose of controls: (1)usual care, or/and rescue medication in consideration of medical ethics; (2) non-insertion sham where the needles do not penetrate the skin, but usually use the blunt end of the acupuncture needles, non-insertion sham devices (e.g. Park sham devices), and other needle-resembling devices such as toothpicks and needling guiding tubes; (3) insertion sham: usually involves a superficial insertion of needles to acupoints or non-acupoints; (4) combined non-insertion and insertion sham; and (5) comparator (positive control): refers to active treatments, such as specific mediations and physiotherapies, some usual care (standardized care), etc., which were thought to be effective. The usual care refers to the standardized patient care in the clinical practices while the individualized cares are available. If a study contained two or more controls types, information on each acupuncture-control comparison pair was extracted according to the control types.

## 2.6.2 Types of Conclusions in Clinical Trials

Positive conclusion was defined as acupuncture showing statistically significant superiority to the control ($p < 0.05$) in the primary outcome of clinical studies. If no primary outcome was stated in the studies, the general conclusion of the study was judged as a positive conclusion when it indicated acupuncture was better than the control.

Negative conclusion was defined as acupuncture not showing statistically significant superiority to the control ($p \geq 0.05$) in the primary outcome of clinical studies. If no primary outcome was stated in the studies, the general conclusion of the article was judged as a negative conclusion if it indicated acupuncture was not better than the control.

An inconclusive conclusion was defined as acupuncture showing statistically significant superiority to the control in some primary outcomes but not in all primary outcomes. If no primary outcome was stated in the studies, the general conclusions of the study was as inconclusive when it indicated acupuncture was somewhat better than the control but not in all outcomes.

## 2.7 Reporting and the Method of Quality Assessment for the References

The quality of the reporting methodology of the included RCTs, were evaluated based on six components from the STRICTA 2010 combined with the Jadad score [155, 156].This modified novel quality assessment tool is named as STRICTA PLUS Scale Score (STRICTA-P) [Table 2.2].

Table2.2: The Novel **STRICTA PLUS** Score components.

| | | STRICTA PLUS Score components |
|---|---|---|
| | **A** | **Jadad Score** |
| | 1 | Was the study described as randomized (this includes words such as randomly, random, and randomization)? |
| | 2 | Was the method used to generate the sequence of randomization described and appropriate (table of random numbers, computer-generated, etc.)? |
| | 3 | Was the study described as double blind? |
| | 4 | Was the method of double blinding described and appropriate (identical placebo, active placebo, dummy, etc.)? |
| | 5 | Was there a description of withdrawals and dropouts? |
| | **B** | **STandards for Reporting Intervention in Controlled Trials of Acupuncture (STRICTA) Guideline** |
| 1 | Acupuncture rationale | 1a) Style of acupuncture (e.g. Traditional Chinese Medicine, Japanese, Korean, Western medical, Five Element, ear acupuncture, etc.) |
| | | 1b) Reasoning for treatment provided, based on historical context, literature sources, and/or consensus methods, with references where appropriate |
| | | 1c) Extent to which treatment was varied |
| 2 | Details of needling | 2a) Number of needle insertions per subject per session (mean and range where relevant) |
| | | 2b) Names (or location if no standard name) of points used (uni/bilateral) |
| | | 2c) Depth of insertion, based on a specified unit of measurement, or on a particular tissue level |
| | | 2d) Response sought (e.g. de qi or muscle twitch response) |
| | | 2e) Needle stimulation (e.g. manual, electrical) |
| | | 2f) Needle retention time |
| | | 2g) Needle type (diameter, length, and manufacturer or material) |
| 3 | Treatment regimen | 3a) Number of treatment sessions |
| | | 3b) Frequency and duration of treatment sessions |
| 4 | Other components of treatment | 4a) Details of other interventions administered to the acupuncture group (e.g. moxibustion, cupping, herbs, exercises, lifestyle advice) |
| | | 4b) Setting and context of treatment, including instructions to practitioners, and information and explanations to patients |
| 5 | Practitioner background | 5) Description of participating acupuncturists (qualification or professional affiliation, years in acupuncture practice, other relevant experience) |
| 6 | Control or comparator interventions | 6a) Rationale for the control or comparator in the context of the research question, with sources that justify this choice |
| | | 6b) Precise description of the control or comparator. If sham acupuncture or any other type of acupuncture-like control is used, provide details as for Items 1 to 3 above. |

## 1. The Jadad Score

The Jadad Score [156] is a tool that is used to assess the quality of randomised controlled trials, specifically in researches related to pain. It is the most cited tool and commonly used scale in the healthcare community. It provides the best validity and reliability evidence, and focuses on three key aspects, namely; randomisation, blinding, and withdrawal or dropout. A score of zero to five is used as a rating, with zero to two score indicating low quality trial and three or above, indicating high quality trials.

Randomisation is a process that helps to prevent factors such as placebo effect or selection bias from interfering with the results of a trial. It allows study groups to be as standardised as possible at baseline, thus aiding to distribute evenly any prognostic factors that may exist. This greatly helps to improve the validity of a study's result. Blinding can be single-blinded or double-blinded. In the case of singled-blinded studies, the assessors and/or participants would not be aware of their group assignment. On the other hand, in a double-blinded study, both the doctors that carry out an intervention, as well as the participants receiving the intervention, would be unaware of their group assignment. The aim of blinding is to reduce the possibility of having the results of a study interfered with personal expectations, placebo and bias that can arise either consciously or subconsciously.

Furthermore, withdrawals refer to any participants who failed to complete an intervention or failed to report data to the researchers. Withdrawals and drop-outs can greatly affect the statistical significance of a study. The five sub-items of the Jadad Score are shown Table 2.2.

## 2. The STandards for Reporting Intervention in Controlled Trials of Acupuncture (STRICTA) Guidelines[2]

The STRICTA, first published in 2001[155], consists of six items and 17 sub-items. This tool helps to assess the completeness and transparency of the way interventions were reported in clinical trials. It outlines the rationale for treatment, needling technique details, treatment regime, additional components of treatment, background of practitioner, control used for the study or comparator interventions (MacPherson et al., 2010) [155].

The 2010 version of the STRICTA guideline is an extension of CONSORT [155]. It is a guideline that helps to improve and highly tune the quality of clinical studies of acupuncture. It makes use of a checklist of six key items, namely; the acupuncture style, the needling details, the treatment protocol, the associated treatments, the acupuncturist background, and the type of control used. The STRICTA guideline items and sub-items are shown in Table: 2.2.

The response used was with either yes or no to each item to judge whether the authors had reported, or had recorded concrete details of the reports accomplished in accordance with the requirement of each item of the checklist of seven key items and 22 sub items of the STRICTA PLUS Scoring Scale (STRICTA-P) quality assessment tool. The responses to some sub-items have been modified due to ambiguity used in some articles in statements refer to these sub-items. Those included (the acupuncturist practitioner background; the setting and context of treatment, including instructions to practitioners, information and explanations to patients; and blindness, etc.). The RCTs' sub items and items which met the standards of the STRICTA-P tool were counted. Thereafter, the corresponding percentage of the application of each item was computed and eventually, the total STRICTA-P score was calculated.

The quality of the 16 selected randomised control trials of this literature review research was assessed using the checklist of the novel tool of STRICTA-P (Table 2.2).

# CHAPTER 3

# RESULTS

## 3.0 Results

A total of sixteen studies were identified and selected using the literature search as defined in the methodology section described before. The studies which have been included in this literature review research are listed in Table 2.1.

The results of this literature review research will be presented under the following two categories:

A. Descriptive summary of the findings; and

B. Analytical review of the included RCTs to assess their strengths and weaknesses.

## 3.1 Descriptive Results

ZHAO Hui-ling and his co-workers in 2007 [157] conducted a study which included sixty patients with DPN who were randomly allocated into two groups of 30 patients each - the acupuncture treated and the control groups. Patients in treatment group were given acupuncture and oral Methycbal (Mecolbalamin) for 8 weeks respectively. The following acu points were used in the management:; Ganshu (BL18), Pishu (BL20), Shenshu (BL23), Feishu (BL13), Yishu, Zusanli (ST36), Sanyinjiao (SP6), Zhaohai (KD6), Quchi(LI11), Hegu (LI4), and Yanglingquan (GB34).In cases diagnosed with Qi and Yin Deficiency, they added Guan Yuan (CV4), and Qi Hai (CV6) point; in those diagnosed with Yin and Yang Deficiency type, they added Qihai (CV6), and Ming Men (GV4) points; and in those diagnosed with blood stasis, they added Geshu (BL17), and Xuehai (SP10) points. The results showed that acupuncture treatment was able to reduce the symptoms and the signs of DPN, decrease whole blood and plasma viscosity, and improve the Nerve Conduction Velocity (NCV) of sensory and motor nerves. The total effective rate of the acupuncture group was 83.33% which was superior to that of the control group (53.33%) and the difference was statistically significant (P<0.01).

Garrow AP and his co-workers in 2014 [158] undertook a RCT that had included 45 DPN patients allocated to receive a 10-week course either of real (53%) or sham (47%) acupuncture. The following five standardized acupuncture points on the lower limb of each leg were used in the study: Tai Chong (LR3),Taxi (KD3), Sanyinjiao (SP6), Xuehai(SP10) and Zusanli (ST36).The

Outcome measures included the Leeds Assessment of Neuropathic Symptoms and Signs (LANSS) scale, lower limb pain (Visual Analogue Scale, VAS); Sleep Problem Scale (SPS); Measure Yourself Medical Outcome Profile (MYMOP); 36-item Short Form 36 Health Survey and resting blood pressure (BP). This trial has demonstrated the applicability and feasibility of acupuncture as an additional treatment for people with DPN. The treatment was highly tolerated with no reported appreciable side effects, however, it concluded that larger randomized trials are needed to further confirm the clinical effectiveness and assess the financial cost of acupuncture in the treatment of DPN.

Lu M. and co-workers in 2016[159] had conducted a study to compare the clinical efficacy between acupuncture and intravenous administration of lipoic acid and alprostadil for DPN. It has included sixty DPN patients who were randomly divided into an acupuncture group (31 cases) and a medication group (29 cases). The main acu points used in this trial were: Geshu (BL17), Ganshu (BL18), Pishu (BL20), Shenshu (Bl23) and Zusanl i(ST36). The following additional points were used in cases with upper limb numbness and pain:Quchi (LI11), Waiguan (SJ5), and Hegu (LI4). In lower limb numbness, the following acupoints were used: Yanglingquan (GB34), Fenglong (ST40), Kunlun (BL60) and Taichong (LR3). Although both acupuncture and conventional medication (control) groups reported satisfaction with the treatment, however, the acupuncture group reported a more marked amelioration in respect to the clinical signs of sensory disorder, reflection disturbance and muscle weakness, nerve conduction and clinical curative effect. The total effective rate was 83.9% (26/31) in the acupuncture group, which was significantly superior to 62.1% (18/29), reported in the medication group (P < 0.05).

Jin Z. and co-workers in 2011[160] conducted a trial to compare the differences in the therapeutic effect on DPN between the combined therapy of electro-acupuncture (EA) and acupoint injection group (A) and the simple acupoint injection (group B). 60 cases of DPN were allocated randomly into these two groups, 30 cases in each one. They had demonstrated that EA and acupoint injection with Methylcobalamin achieve a significant clinical therapeutic efficacy on DPN with an efficacy that was significantly higher to that of simple management with acupoint injection with Methylcobalamin. The EA plus injection group selected acupoints were:Gongsun (SP4) through Yongquan (KD1) through Taichong (LR 3), Taixi (KD3) through the Kunlun (BL60), Sanyinjiao (SP6) through Xuan Zhong (GB39), Yin Ling Quan (SP9) through Yang Ling Quan (GB34), Quchi (LI11)through Xiao Hai (SI8). This trial had demonstrated that EA can effectively increase nerve conduction velocity, control and relieve the symptoms of DPN. In EA plus acupoint injection group (group A), EA and acupoint injection with Methylcobalamin were administered. Penetrating acupuncture was mainly applied from Gongsun (SP 4) to Quanzhong (Extra) and from Yongquan (KI 1) to Taichong (LR 3). Acupoint injection was administered on Sanyinjiao (SP 6). In the acupoint injection group (group B), only acupoint injection with Methylcobalamin was provided on the Sanyinjiao (SP 6) point. Following two sessions of treatment, the conduction velocity of ulnar nerve and tibial nerves were measured. The scores of the Chinese medicine syndrome and the DPN were recorded before and after treatment in two groups. The effective rates were 90.0% (27/30) and 63.3% (19/30) in group A and group B respectively, presenting significant statistical difference (P < 0.05). After treatment, the motor nerve conduction velocity (MCV) and sensory nerve conduction velocity (SCV) of ulnar nerve and tibial nerve in group A were significantly superior to those in group B (P < 0.05, P < 0.01).

Ji XQ. And co-workers in a 2010 study [161] investigated the effect of acupuncture treatment on the nerve conduction function in patients with DPN by assessing the effect of spleen-stomach regulation-needling on the nerve conduction activity in patients with DPN. It included eighty patients with DPN who were equally randomized into an acupuncture group and a medication group – 40 patients in each group. Patients in the medication group were treated with intramuscular injection of Mecobalamine (500 microg) once daily for 4 weeks. The SCV, MCV, the amplitude and latency of the evoked potential of the tibial nerve were detected before and after the treatment by using an Electromyography and Evoked Potential Equipment. In the acupuncture group, the following acupuncture points were used: Quchi (LI11), Hegu (LI4), Zhongwan (CV12), Xuehai (SP10), Diji (SP8), Zusanli (ST36), Yin Lingquan (SP9), Yang Lingquan(GB34) and Sanyinjiao (SP6) points. After the treatment, the total effective reported rates were 82.5% and 95.0% respectively. This confirmed that acupuncture for regulating spleen-stomach function might have a better effect on the conduction function of the tibial nerve than Mecobalamine in the treatment of diabetic patients with DPN.

Tong Y and co-workers in 2010 [162] investigated the effects of acupuncture on DPN. They compared 42 cases treated using the acupuncture with 21 cases exposed to sham acupuncture and observed the effects on nerve conduction velocity and a variety of subjective symptoms associated with DPN. A total of 10 acupoints were used in this study: Hegu (LI4), Fenglong (ST40), Quchi (LI11), Zusanli (ST36), and Sanyinjiao (SP6) points. These points were identified by an experienced acupuncturist according to traditional methods. Three of the six measures of motor nerves and two measures of sensory function demonstrated significant improvement (p < 0.05) over a 15-day treatment period in the acupuncture group, while no motor or sensory function was significantly improved in the sham acupuncture group. There were also significant differences in vibration perception threshold between the groups (p < 0.05) and when compared to the baseline levels (p < 0.01) in the acupuncture group. Accordingly, they concluded that the real acupuncture was significantly more effective compared to the sham acupuncture for treatment of numbness of the lower extremities, spontaneous pain in the lower extremities, rigidity in the upper extremities and alterations in temperature perception in the lower extremities(different symptoms of DPN) after therapy. This pilot study has, therefore, provided evidence that acupuncture may be clinically useful for the radical treatment of DPN.

Zhang C and co-workers in 2010 undertook a study [163] to observe the clinical effects of acupuncture for DPN. The study included 65 patients who were randomly divided into a treatment group of 32 cases and a control group of 33 cases. The main points selected were: Ganshu (BL 18), Pishu (BL 20), Shenshu (BL 23), Yishu, Feishu (BL 58), Zusanli (ST 36), Sanyinjiao (SP 6), Taibai (SP 3), Zutonggu (BL 66), Qihai (CV 6), Guanyuan (CV 4), Fenglong (ST 40) and Yanglingquan (GB 34) points. The auxiliary points used in cases diagnosed with blood stasis were: Jianyu (LI 15), Quchi (LI 11), Shousanli (LI 10), Hegu (LI 4), Biguan (ST 31), Futu (ST 32), Liangqiu (ST 34), Xiangu (ST 43) and Neiting (ST 44). Xuehai (SP 10) and Geshu (BL 17); while the Yinlingquan (SP 9) and Diji (SP 8) points were added for phlegm; and Bafeng (EX-LE10) and Baxie (EX-UE9) points were added for severe numbness of the hands and feet. On the basis of conventional treatment of diabetes, acupuncture was used in the treatment group while inositol was orally administered in the control group. During a 3-month treatment regimen, changes in the symptomatology were observed and recorded. The total effective rates were of 87.5% and of 63.6%.in acupuncture and control group respectively which is taken as evidence based indication that acupuncture can show positive effects for treatment of DPN.

Chen YL. And co-workers in 2009 [164] conducted a RCT to assess the effects of penetrating acupuncture on peripheral nerve conduction velocity in patients with DPN. This study included 71 patients with DPN who were divided into acupuncture group (n = 38) and mecobalamin (control) group (n = 33) using simple random method based on the random number table and card count. Acupuncture treatment was given once a day for 12 times and oral Mecobalamin treatment administered at a dose of 0.5 mg, three times daily for 12 days after which the efficacy was evaluated in both groups. In the acupuncture group, the chosen acupuncture points were: YinlingQuan (SP9), YangLingQuan (GB34), Neiguan (PC6) through Waiguan (SJ5), and Zusanli (ST36), Sanyinjiao (SP6), Geshu (BL17), and Shenshu (BL23). On EA, acupuncture was done on YinLingquan (SP9) and Zusanli (ST36) acupoints. The results demonstrated improvement of NCV in lower extremity of DPN patients which was better than that of oral administration of mecobalamin in the control group. However, there was no significant difference between the two groups in improving the conduction velocity of upper limb nerve. This latter observation was explained by the fact that it might be related to the use of EA in the lower limbs but not in the upper limbs! Accordingly, they have emphasized and suggested that the EA is to be considered in the future study because of its possible potential role to improve the patient's neurological function.

Jiang H and co-workers in a trial conducted in 2006 [165] set out to examine the mechanisms of wrist-ankle acupuncture for prevention and treatment of DPN. It included ninety cases of DPN who were randomly divided into 3 groups of 30 patients each (Group I, group II and group III) being treated respectively with wrist-ankle acupuncture, body-acupuncture, and the western routine medical treatment. The clinical therapeutic effects and laboratory results were then compared between the groups. Group I was treated with wrist-ankle acupuncture. For Group II, in which body acupuncture was used, the local points combined with the symptomatologic points were selected which included the following: Sanyinjiao (SP6), Xuehai (SP10), Taixi (KI3), Quchi (LI11), and Yanglingquan (GB34); the points of the upper limb: Jianyu (LI15), Jianliao (SJ14), Quchi (LI11), Waiguan (SJ5), and Hegu (LI4);and the points on the lower limb: Huantiao (GB30), Zusanli (ST36), Yanglingquan (GB34), Jiexi (ST41), and Neiting (ST44). For the type of stagnation of *qi* and blood stasis, Xingjian (LR2) and Xuehai (SP10) points were added; for the damp-heat type, Dazhui (GV14) and Neiguan (PC6) points were added; and for the type of deficiency of blood due to cold, moxibustion on Geshu (BL17), Pishu (BL20) and Zusanli (ST36) points were added. Although there were significant differences between the two acupuncture groups, the results indicated that the therapeutic effects of the wrist-ankle acupuncture group and the body acupuncture group were significantly superior to those of the control group and these outcomes gave a scientific evidence that the Wrist-ankle acupuncture has the actions of improving the metabolisms in diabetic patients, and potentially restoring the functions of peripheral nerve cells, thus giving positive therapeutic effects for DPN. The comparison of the therapeutic results of the three Groups demonstrated that the total effective rates of Group I and Group II are obviously superior to that of Group III. The decreasing rate of the total evaluation score for the clinical symptoms after the treatment was 75% in Group I, 73% in Group II, obviously higher than 59% of Group III, pointing out that wrist-ankle acupuncture and body acupuncture can significantly improve the clinical symptoms and raise the therapeutic effects. Furthermore, the comparison of the conductive velocity of limb motor nerve of the 3 Groups, demonstrated significant improvement in the NCV of Group I and Group II ($P<0.05$ or $P<0.01$), with the functions improved; but there was no obvious improvement in Group III, indicating that wrist-ankle acupuncture and body acupuncture can positively ameliorate the nerve functions in patients with DPN.

Anne Bailey and her co-workers in 2017 [166] had undertaken a study aimed at assessing the effectiveness of the acupuncture treatment for DPN symptoms and lower extremity arterial circulation in people with type 2 diabetes (T2DM). Twenty-five patients, who reported a threshold level of the DPN symptoms in the lower extremities during 4 weeks before the beginning of the study, had received acupuncture treatment once per week over a 10-week period. The Neuropathy Total Symptom Scale (NTSS-6), Neuropathy Disability Score (NDS), and laser Doppler fluxmetry (LDF) were used for assessment the effectiveness of the acupuncture treatment at baseline and 10 weeks. The commonly selected acu points included: Futu (ST32), Shangjuxu (ST37), Chongyang (ST42), Lougu (SP7), Yinlinqguan (SP9), Yongquan (KD1), Taixi (KD3), Zhubin (KD9), Zhongfeng (LR4), Xiguan (LR7), Yanglinqguan (GB34), Guangming (GB37), and the Bafeng points. A total of 19 of 25 study participants completed the study and reported a significant reduction in the NTSS symptoms of aching pain, burning pain, prickling sensation, numbness, and allodynia. The lancinating pain did not decrease significantly. The LDF measures improved but not significantly. The conclusion was that the acupuncture may effectively improve selected DPN symptoms in these American Indian patients. In this particular study, the concept of random allocation to the treatment group was not well-received in this community, with the majority of eligible and willing candidates agreeing to participation contingent on inclusion into the acupuncture treatment group. This eventually resulted that the study had only one-group design which limits statistical analysis to within-group before and after comparisons, rather than the between-groups longitudinal analysis that was in the original design. This constitutes a substantial loss of the statistical power and the robustness of this trial as treatment group results could not be compared with the natural fluctuation in DPN symptoms that may occur with the usual care. However, the LDF measures of endothelial functioning did increase over the study period (10 week), with a mean 18% increase in endothelial-dependent and a 26% increase in endothelial independent vasodilatation which was not statistically significant. It is important to note that the LDF measures tend to have a high statistical variance which as a result would require larger samples sizes to detect greater than chance differences.

SUN Yuan-zheng and XU Ying-yingin 2010 [167] conducted a RCT aimed to observe the clinical therapeutic efficacy of warm acupuncture in the treatment of DPN and its effects on the conduction velocity of the tibial nerve and common fibular nerve. Fifty-two subjects were equally randomized into two groups and treated by conventional therapy. In addition, the control group was given mecobalamin injection at 500 μg, once a day for four weeks, while the treatment group was given warm acupuncture, 6 times a week for 4 weeks. The chosen Acupoints were: Pishu (BL 20), Shenshu (BL 23), Huantiao (GB 30), Zusanli (ST 36), Yanglingquan (GB 34), Sanyinjiao (SP 6), Taixi (KD 3), Quchi(LI 11), Waiguan (SJ 5), and Hegu (LI 4) acupoints. The clinical efficacy and the NCV of the tibial nerve and common fibular nerve were observed and compared between the two groups. After four-week treatments, the total effective rate in acupuncture group was 88.5% which was significantly higher than 61.5% in the control group (P<0.05). The conduction velocity of tibial nerve and common fibular nerve was higher in both groups (P<0.05), with higher conduction velocity in the acupuncture group (P<0.05). These results demonstrated that warm acupuncture is quite effective to treat and improve nerve conduction velocity in patients with DPN.

Wang Hui and co-workers in 2015 [168] conducted a RCT to compare the efficacy of two different acupuncture (total therapy, topical therapy) in the treatment of DPN, in order to guide the optimization of clinical treatment. Sixty seven patients with DPN were included in this study and were randomly divided into treatment group and control group. The used head and body acupoints were the following: Baihui(GV20), Sishencong (Ex), Guan Yuan (CV4),Qihai (CV6), the Feng Chi (GB20), Geshu (BL17), Ganshu (BL18), and Shenshu (Bl23); limbs Acupoints treatment: selection of meridians based on the meridian theory, upper limb acupoints; Quchi (LI11), Waiguan (SJ5), Ba Xie (On the Hand), lower extremity acupoints; Zusanli (ST36), Taixi (KD3), Zhaohai (KD6), Bafeng (Ex) 4 points on each foot. Nerve conduction studies were used to monitor the MNCV of the median nerve, ulnar nerve and peroneal nerve of the bilateral limbs before and after treatment, and SNCV changes, analysis and comparison of its clinical treatment. The total effective rate was 89.7% in the treatment group, which was significantly (P<0.05) higher than that in the control group (64.9%). The results illustrated that when acupuncture and moxibustion therapies in whole body (Extremities and trunk) were used in combination to treat DPN, overall therapy is superior to the local peripheral acupuncture treatment.

Zhao Zhixuan and co-workers in a 2010 [169] study observed the clinical treatment effect of the application of the combined scalp and body acupuncture techniques in the treatment of DPN. It included 78 cases of DPN who were randomly allocated to the treatment group and to the control group. The two groups received a 30 day-course of treatment. The selected Body acupoints were: Quchi (LI11), Waiguan (SJ5), Hegu (LI4), Zusanli (ST36), Yanglingquan (GB34), Xuan Zhong (alt. JueGu) GB39, and Taichong (LR3).The Scalp acupoints were: Babel back to lead the 1.5-inch line (double Side), is back to lead a long 1.5-inch line to Cheng Ling (GB18) bilateral. The total reported effective rate was 91% in the treatment group and 66.7% in the control group and there was significant difference between the two groups (P <0.05). There was a significant difference in the overall tests of the NCV before and after treatment in both groups compared with the control group P <0.05. These clinically and statistically significant results proved that the scalp acupuncture with body acupuncture can help in the treatment of DPN.

FEI Ai-hua and co-workers conducted a study in 2011[170] to assess the acupuncture clinical therapeutic effect on DPN and its impact on inflammatory cytokine-hypersensitive C-reactive protein (hs-CRP). Sixty patients with DPN were randomly distributed between the treatment and the control groups. In addition to basic treatment for diabetes, Mecobalamin was given to the control group and acupuncture was done to the treatment group. The selected acupoints were the following: Geshu (BL17), Shenshu (BL23), Yishu, Zusanli (ST36) and Sanyinjiao (SP6).The clinical symptoms, MNCV and SNCV, and hs-CRP were examined in the two groups before and after treatment. The results illustrated that the total efficacy rate in the treatment group of 90% was significantly higher than that in the control group of 60% ($P<0.05$). After the acupuncture treatment, the nerve conduction velocity increased markedly ($P<0.01$) and hs-CRP decreased significantly ($P<0.01$). These promising results lead to the conclusion that acupuncture treatment has a promising positive therapeutic effect on DPN and can lower hs-CRP levels.

GAO Yu in 2016 undertook a study [171] with the objective of investigating the clinical effect of the acupuncture and the moxibustion in the treatment of DPN. It included ninety patients with DPN who were randomly allocated into two groups. The acupuncture group who was treated with conventional treatment combined with acupuncture treatment while the control group was treated with conventional treatment. The upper limb selected acupoints were: Jianliao (SJ14), Quchi (LI11), Waiguan (SJ5) and Hegu (LI4);the lower limb acupoints were: Yanglinqguan (GB34), Zusanli (ST36), Taichong (LV3) and Zhao hai(KD6). The total effective rate in the acupuncture group was 86.67%, which was significantly higher than that of the control group

71.11% (P<0.05). This RCT demonstrated that acupuncture and moxibustion treatments have high clinical efficacy for DPN and are worthy of application and promotion.

ZUO Lin and ZHANG Lin in 2010 [172] undertook a study aimed to investigate the effects of acupuncture plus methylcobalamin in treating DPN. Seventy-five with DPN were included and randomly allocated into a treatment group (40 cases) and a control group (35 cases). The patients in the treatment group all have given acupuncture therapy plus methylcobalamin. The patients in the control group were given only methylcobalamin for treatment. The therapeutic effect was evaluated four weeks later. The selected acupoints were: Bilateral Zusanli (ST 36), Sanyinjiao (SP 6), Taixi (KD 3), Quchi (LI 11), Hegu (LI 4), Waiguan (SJ 5), as well as Guanyuan (CV 4) and Qihai (CV 6).The results of the used evaluation indices demonstrated statistically significant improvement of symptoms and physical signs of the study population. In the acupuncture group, the effective rate of 90.0% was superior to that in the control group of 77.1% and the difference was statistically significant (P<0.05). The difference of the nervous system score between pre-treatment and post-treatment of the treatment group was also statistically significant (P<0.001). Furthermore, after treatment, the MNCV and SNCV of median and peroneal nerves of the treatment group was markedly faster than that of pre-treatment (P<0.01), and it had a significant increase compared with the control group (P<0.01). These results demonstrated the positive effects of acupuncture therapy in patients with DPN.

## 3.2 Analytical Results

### 3.2.1 Results of the STRICTA PLUS Scoring Scale (STRICTA-P)

The included RCT's in this literature review study were assessed using the novel STRICTA-P score as described in the Methodology section. This score allows for a standardized assessment of quality control of the various studies with the ideal score being a total of 22. The STRICTA-P results relevant to the studies in question are shown in table 3.1.

**Table3.1: Results of the total score of STRICTA PLUS Scoring Scale (STRICTA-P).**

| | Study name and date | Jadad Score (5) | STRICTA* Guidelines | Acupuncture rationale (3) | Details of needling (7) | Treatment regimen (2) | Other components of treatment (2) | Practitioner background (1) | Control or comparator interventions (2) | Total STRICTA PLUS SCORE (STRICTA-P)(22) |
|---|---|---|---|---|---|---|---|---|---|---|
| 1 | ZHAO Hui-ling , et al. 2007 [157] | 1 | | 3 | 3.5 | 2 | 1 | 0 | 2 | 12.5 |
| 2 | Garrow AP., et al 2014 [158] | 2 | | 3 | 7 | 2 | 2 | 1 | 2 | 19 |
| 3 | Lu M., et al. 2016 [159] | 2 | | 3 | 5.5 | 2 | 2 | 0 | 2 | 16.5 |
| 4 | Jin Z., et al 2011 [160] | 2 | | 3 | 6.5 | 2 | 1 | 0 | 2 | 16.5 |
| 5 | Ji XQ., et al 2010 [161] | 2 | | 3 | 7 | 2 | 2 | 0 | 2 | 18 |
| 6 | Tong Y., et al. 2010 [162] | 2 | | 3 | 7 | 2 | 2 | 0 | 2 | 18 |
| 7 | Zhang C., et al, 2010 [163] | 2 | | 3 | 7 | 2 | 2 | 0.5 | 2 | 18.5 |
| 8 | Chen YL., et al 2009 [164] | 2 | | 3 | 7 | 2 | 2 | 0 | 2 | 18 |
| 9 | Jiang H, et al. 2006 [165] | 2 | | 3 | 7 | 2 | 2 | 0 | 2 | 18 |
| 10 | Anne Bailey., et al 2017 [166] | 2 | | 3 | 7 | 2 | 2 | 0 | 1 | 17 |
| 11 | SUN Y-Z, XU Y-y. 2010 [167] | 2 | | 3 | 7 | 2 | 2 | 0 | 2 | 18 |
| 12 | Wang Hui, et al 2015 [168] | 1 | | 3 | 6 | 2 | 1.5 | 0 | 2 | 15.5 |
| 13 | Zhao Zhixuan, et al. 2010 [169] | 1 | | 3 | 6 | 2 | 1 | 0 | 2 | 15 |
| 14 | FEI Ai-hua, et al 2011 [170] | 1 | | 3 | 4 | 2 | 0 | 0 | 2 | 12 |
| 15 | GAO Yu 2016 [171] | 2 | | 3 | 4 | 2 | 1 | 0 | 2 | 14 |
| 16 | ZUO Lin, ZHANG Lin 2010 [172] | 1 | | 3 | 5.5 | 2 | 1 | 0 | 2 | 14.5 |

The average STRICTA-P Score for all the studies is 16.31 (74.2%), the minimum STRICTA-P score is 12 [171] (54.6%) and maximum STRICTA-P score is 19 [158] (86.4%).

## 3.2.2 Other analytical results

### 3.2.2.1 Population

The total study population of the selected studies was approximately 1070. The minimum average age of the population in all the included studies was 43.5 ± 5.0 years in the acupuncture group [162]. The maximum average age of the population in the selected trials was 68.55 ± 8.91 years in acupuncture group [164].

### 3.2.2.2 Diagnostic Criteria in the Selected Trials

Variable diagnostic criteria for Diabetes and DPN have been implemented in the analyzed RCTs and quarter of the selected studies failed to refer to any diagnostic criteria.

**The Diabetes Diagnostic criteria used in the selected studies are the following:**

➤ 7 studies [160, 161, 163-165, 167, 170] (43.75%) used the WHO 1999 diagnostic criteria [154].

➤ Two trials [169, 172] (12.5%) have applied the American Diabetes Association (ADA) 1997 diagnostic criteria [173].

➤ One trial [171] (6.25%) applied the Chinese Medical Association Diabetes Branch diagnostic criteria.

➤ One trial [157] (6.25%) has adopted western criteria with reference to Shen Zhaoyuan editor of the diabetes Chronic complications [174] and Jiang Yu-ping editor of the clinical neurological disease [175].

➤ Five RCTs [158, 159, 162, 166, 168] (31.25%) failed to specify any diagnostic criteria.

**The DPN Diagnostic criteria used in the selected RCTs:**

➤ One trial [170] (6.25%) applied the WHOPNTF on DPN diagnostic criteria.

➤ Two trials [157, 165] (12.5%) have applied the Chinese Medical Association Diabetes Branch diagnostic criteria with reference to the Diagnostic Criteria drawn by Qian Zhaoren [176] in which TCM differentiation was done in accordance with the criteria set by Lin Lan [177].

➤ One trial [161] (6.25%) implemented the Japanese simple diagnostic criteria of DPN which was revised on 2002 [178].

➤ The majority of the analyzed trials (eight RCTs which constitute 50% of the total included RCTs) [158, 160, 163, 164, 166, 167, 169, 172] had given the description of symptoms and the signs of DPN without specifying any diagnostic criteria.

## 3.2.2.3 Control Groups

Various types of controls were selected in the analyzed RCT's and included the following;

> Two trials (12.5%) used Sham control [158, 162].

> Methycobalamin was used in different forms (oral, Intravenous, intramuscular and in acupoint injection)

  • Oral mecobalamin (tablet of 0.5 mg) was used in three studies (18.75%) [157, 164, 170].

  • One study (6.25%) used Acupoint injection of methylcobalamin [160].

  • Two trials (12.5%) used intra muscular mecocobalamin in the control groups [161, 167].

  • One trial (6.25%) used intramuscular injection of $VitB_1$ 100mg, $VitB_{12}$ 500μg in control group [169].

  • Intravenous methylcobalamin 500μg once a day was used by one trial [172] (6.25%).

> One study [163] (6.25%) had used oral inositol (2gm per day in three times) in the control group.

> One trial [159] (6.25%) used intravenous lipoic acid (0.6gm) and Alprastadil (10mg) in the control group.

> Two trials [165, 171] (12.5%) used the usual western medical care in the control groups.

## 3.2.2.4 Duration of Diabetes and DPN

The Diabetes as well as the DPN duration in the population of the selected trials is illustrated in table 3.1. DPN duration in acupuncture groups had ranged from 2.1±0.63 in trial of Tong Y., et al. 2010 [162] to 5.64± 4.77 in Jiang H, et al. 2006 [165] study (wrist ankle acu group);however, in the control groups, it ranged from 1.96±0.67 years in Tong Y., et al. 2010 [162] to 5.81 ± 4.38 years in Jiang H, et al. 2006 [165].Nevertheless, the duration of diabetes in acupuncture groups had a wider range as it ranges from 2.53±0.53 years in Wang Hui, et al 2015[168] to 12.67±1.3 in Tong Y, Guo H, Han B. 2010 [162]. In the control groups, the diabetes duration ranged from 2.96 ± 0.49in Wang Hui, et al 2015[168] to 12.4±1.3 years in Tong Y., et al. 2010[162].

Table3.2: Data about the duration of Diabetes, DPN and the total efficacy rates of the investigated studies-(Acu* Gp=Acupuncture Group, C- Gp=Control Group).

| No | Authors | Study Groups | Total efficacy rate (%) | Duration of diabetes (Years) | Duration of DPN (Years) |
|---|---|---|---|---|---|
| 1 | ZHAO Huiling , et al. 2007 [157] | Acu* Gp | 83.33% | 9.91 ± 5.28 | 2.71 ± 2.58 |
| | | C- Gp | 53.33%. | | |
| 2 | Garrow AP., et al.2014[158] | Acu* Gp | Thirteen of 24 (46.4%) showed at least a 25% improvement in VAS pain intensity score. | 11.0 ±9.2 | |
| | | C- Gp (Sham) | compared with four of 21 (12.9%) in the sham treatment group. | 12.2 (7.4) | |
| 3 | Lu M., et al. 2016 [159] | Acu* Gp | 83.9% | | 3.6±1.3 |
| | | C- Gp | 62.1% | | 3.5±1.1 |
| 4 | Jin Z., et al 2011 [160] | Acu* Gp | 90.0 %(27/30) | 7.30 ± 4.21 | 3.12 ± 1.23 |
| | | C- Gp | 63 .3% (19/30) | 7.28 ± 3.65 | 3.15 ± 1.12 |
| 5 | Ji XQ., et al 2010 [161] | Acu* Gp | 95.0% | 9.45 ± 2.73 | 3.77 ± 1.16 |
| | | C- Gp | 82.5% | 8.70 ± 2.95 | 3.44 ± 1.29 |
| 6 | Tong Y, Guo H, Han B. 2010 [162] | Acu* Gp | In the acupuncture group, three of the six measures in motor nerves demonstrated significant improvement ($p<0.05$) over the 15-day treatment period. | 12.67±1.3 | 2.1±0.63 |
| | | C Gp (Sham) | | 12.4±1.3 | 1.96±0.67 |
| 7 | Zhang C, Ma YX, Yan Y. 2010 [163] | Acu* Gp | 87.5%. | | 1–5 years. |
| | | C Gp | 63.6%. | | 0.5–5 years. |

| No | Authors | Study Groups | Total efficacy rate (%) | | Duration of diabetes (Years) | Duration of DPN (Years) |
|---|---|---|---|---|---|---|
| 8 | Chen YL., et al 2009 [164] | Acu* Gp | The effect of acupuncture on the motor nerve conduction velocity and the sensory nerve conduction velocity of the common peroneal nerve was significantly better than that of mecobalamin (P<0.05). | | 12.06 ± 7.69 | 2.23 ± 1.52 |
|  |  | C-Gp (mecobalamin) |  | |  |  |
| 9 | Jiang H, et al. 2006 [165] | Acu*Gp1 (wrist-ankle acupuncture) | 93.39% | |  | 5.64± 4.77 |
|  |  | Acu* Gp II (body-acupuncture) | 90.00% | |  | 5.49 ± 4.32 |
|  |  | C-Gp(usual western care Gp) | 63.33% | |  | 5.81 ± 4.38 |
| 10 | Anne Bailey., et al 2017[166] | Acu* Gp | Complete | 19 | 12± 7 |  |
|  |  |  | Incomplete | 6 | 16±14 |  |
| 11 | SUN Yuan-zheng, XU Ying-ying. 2010 [167] | Acu* Gp | 88.5% | | 7.13±5.22 | 2.47±1.74 |
|  |  | C Gp | 61.5% | | 6.78±5.39 | 2.46±1.99 |
| 12 | Wang Hui, et al 2015 [168] | Acu* Gp | 89.7%. | |  | 2.53±0.53 |
|  |  | C Gp | 64.9% | |  | 2.96 ± 0.49 |
| 13 | Zhao Zhixuan, et al. 2010 [169] | Acu* Gp | 91% | | 6.0 | 2.4 |
|  |  | C Gp | 66.7% | | 6.5 | 2.5 |
| 14 | FEI Ai-hua, et al 2011 [170] | Acu* Gp | 90% | | 10.1 ± 0.5 | 2.43 ± 0.23 |
|  |  | C Gp | 60% | | 10.33 ± 0.42 | 2.53 ± 0.28 |
| 15 | GAO Yu 2016 [171] | Acu* Gp | 86.67 | |  | 4.53 ± 1.26 |
|  |  | C Gp | 71.11% | |  | 4.23 ± 1.13 |
| 16 | ZUO Lin, ZHANG Lin 2010 [172] | Acu* Gp | 90.0%. | | 8.7 |  |
|  |  | C Gp | 77.1%. | | 8.5 |  |

### 3.2.2.5 Acupuncture Intervention

All the studies (100%) used the Traditional Chinese style of acupuncture and for locating the selected the acupoints. While the majority of the trials conducted the manual needle stimulation, two studies [160, 168] (12.5%) combined the manual acupuncture with the electrical acupuncture; and one study [167] (6.25%) used the warm acupuncture (acupuncture with moxabustion). Furthermore, while most of the trials had conducted body acupuncture, two studies [168, 169] (12.5%) used the scalp acupuncture in addition to the body acupuncture in the treatment groups[169] and one study (6.25%) used the Wrist-Ankle acupuncture [165] as a separate study group in addition to the body acupuncture and the control groups.

### 3.2.2.6 Outcomes and Efficacy Rates

The total efficacy rates are illustrated in table 3.2. The results shows clearly that the total efficacy rates in acupuncture treatment groups ranged from 83.33% in ZHAO Hui-ling et al.(2007)[157] to 95% in Ji XQ.et al (2010) [161] and the total efficacy rates in control groups ranged from 53.33% in ZHAO Hui-ling et al.(2007) [157] to 77.1% in ZUO Lin and ZHANG Lin (2010) [172].

### 3.2.2.7 Reporting Blinding Process, Adverse Effects and Drop Outs

Although most of studies showed concordance between the number of the recruited population and the final results figures, however they failed to report clearly the withdrawal rates, the adverse effects and blinding process. The exceptions to this were the following studies;

➢        Garrow AP. et al (2014) [158], was the only study which reported in details the withdrawal from the trial. It included the information in the study design under adverse event reporting section which stated that at the beginning of each study visit. Patients were asked if they had had any side effects as a result of the acupuncture treatment. Furthermore, patients were given with a telephone number to report any concerns they had about the study. Any adverse events were recorded on the case report forms and reported to the principal investigator and the research and development department according to the hospital's standard operating procedures. All patients with suspected adverse events received a referral appointment with the study principal investigator - a consultant in diabetes - to determine whether the event was related to the acupuncture treatment.

The reported adverse events were as follows; three adverse events resulted in patients withdrawing from the trial. Two were from the acupuncture group and one from sham acupuncture group.

The forms of these effects were as follows; in the group receiving real acupuncture treatment, one participant developed chest pains while undergoing acupuncture treatment, which was related to a chronic heart condition, and another withdrew because she felt that the acupuncture exacerbated her leg pain. In the sham group, one participant withdrew because she developed a localized swelling in her leg, which was considered unrelated to the study. However, no cases of infections associated with the administration of acupuncture were seen or reported. Furthermore; Garrow AP. et al (2014) [158] reported clearly as single-blind, placebo-controlled RCT.

➢   Lu M, et al. (2016)[159] only pointed briefly that no adverse reactions without any further details in the design and results of the study literature, however it did not provide any information about the dropout rate and the blinding procedure.


➢   Tong Y. et al. (2010) [162] reported the blinding data comprehensively in the results section. By using the blinding indices, 0.32 (95% CI, 0.27 to 0.37) in the acupuncture group and −0.65 (95% CI, −0.61 to −0.69) in the sham acupuncture group, the researchers showed that 32% of patients correctly guessed the treatment identity beyond chance, while 65% of patients in the sham acupuncture group incorrectly guessed that they had received acupuncture. However, after assessing these results, the trial investigators indicated high "response bias", which implied that most of the study participants tend to believe that they were assigned to a more effective intervention.

➤ Anne Bailey.et al (2017) [166] although reporting briefly that there were no adverse events from the acupuncture treatment, the results had shown that six participants among the 25 in the treatment group did not complete the course of acupuncture. They further explained that the most prominent reason for dropping out of the study was the concerns with other diabetes co morbidities, as those who did not complete the treatment were more likely to have cardiovascular disease, nephropathy, peripheral vascular disease, and/or retinopathy. Anne Bailey.et al (2017) [166] did not report the blinding process.

➤ ZUO Lin and ZHANG Lin (2010) [172] in the final part of the discussion section, they have reported briefly that the trial did not show any adverse effect.

Therefore, only four studies [158, 159, 166, 172] which constitute 25% of the selected studies have reported the adverse effects of the acupuncture and the sham treatments; two studies [158, 166] which constitute 12.5% of the tested trials had reported the dropout rates and the reasons of those withdrawals; and only two studies [158, 162] which constitute 12.5% of the tested RCTs had reported and explained the blinding data.

# CHAPTER 4

# DISCUSSION

## 4.0 Discussion

DPN is common disease that has been managed by acupuncture treatment. In Malta, such a complimentary therapeutic option is not currently available and a review of the relevant available literature may build up sufficient evidence to enable acupuncture to be introduced as a complimentary therapeutic option in cases of DPN. In this literature review, a total of about thirteen RCT databases were systemically researched and analyzed for study strength. A new assessment tool – STRICTA Plus Scoring Scale (STRICTA-P) – was used in this study to assess the quality of the used methodology and standard data reporting of the included RCTs. The STRICTA-P tool includes an amalgamation of the STRICTA statement which is the most widely accepted specific technical standards for reporting quality assessment in acupuncture studies [155], and the Jadad Score [156] which is a tool that is used to assess the general quality parameters of the RCTs and it is the most cited and the most commonly used RCTs assessment tool in the healthcare community. The use of STRICTA-P tool is one of the main strength of this literature review study.

This literature review showed that acupuncture treatment might be a useful, effective and potentially safe complementary therapeutic tool in the management of DPN. However, these positive finding should be interpreted cautiously and conservatively, due to the fact that all the included trials suffer from a high risk of bias, the possibility of publication bias, and the major variability of the used acupuncture protocols. Therefore, because of the relative poor methodological quality of the included trials, this review was not able to provide concrete conclusive evidence about the therapeutic effect of the acupuncture for DPN. This applies to the therapeutic use of manual acupuncture, electro-acupuncture, moxibustion, trunk acupuncture, upper and lower extremities acupuncture, wrist and ankle acupuncture as well as scalp acupuncture.

In this study, all the included RCTs were evaluated as high risk of bias, which also has been the strategy in a few numbers of previous reviews [181, 182, 183]. Furthermore, the poor methodology of the majority of the included trials prohibited the conduction of a meaningful sensitivity analysis as planned.

It was not possible to determine the robustness of the results of this review due to the exclusion of the trials with inadequate methodology and in spite of that, still the majority of the included trials were of relatively poor methodology [181].

Application of the novel STRICTA PLUS Scale Score (STRICTA-P) is considered to be one of the strengths of this study and its' average was 16.31 (74.15%), with the minimum STRICTA-P score of 12 [171] (54.55%) and the maximum STRICTA-P score of 19 [158] (86.36%). Nevertheless, dissecting the STRICTA-P results, shows that most of the included trials failed to achieve 50% rate of the five points Jadad score as eleven trials (Garrow AP., et al 2014 [158], Lu M., et al. 2016 [159], Jin Z., et al 2011[160], Ji XQ., et al 2010 [161], Tong Y., et al. 2010 [162], Zhang C., et al, 2010 [163], Chen YL., et al 2009 [164], Jiang H, et al. 2006 [165], Anne Bailey., et al 2017 [166], SUN Y-Z, XU Y-y. 2010[167], and GAO Yu 2016 [171] ) have scored 2 (40%) out of the total 5 points and five trials (ZHAO Hui-ling , et al. 2007 [157], Wang Hui, et al 2015 [168] , Zhao Zhixuan, et al. 2010 [169] , FEI Ai-hua, et al 2011[17] and ZUO Lin, ZHANG Lin 2010[172]) scored 1 (20%) out of 5.

In addition to this, the majority of the tested RCTs (87.5%) scored zero for the Practitioner background score of (1) and only one study (Garrow AP., et al 2014 [158]) scored 1 (100%) and another study (Zhang C., et al, 2010 [163]) scored 0.5 (50%) [Table3.2]. Nevertheless, the other scoring parameters of the novel STRICTA-P tool were relatively on average well scored in the analyzed reviews. These facts reflect the relative poor quality of the methodology of the included trials.

A total of 63 potentially relevant articles were retrieved during this literature search. Of these, 47 studies were excluded because they did not meet the predetermined selection criteria. Eventually, sixteen studies which met the inclusion criteria and provided exclusive information about the use of acupuncture for treatment of DPN were chosen and were included in this literature review (Table.2.1)-(Figure: 2.1). The total population of the selected sixteen studies of this literature review meta-analysis were approximately 1070 (average about 67 participants per study) which represents a small study population that might significantly lower the power of these RCTs. None of the included analysed trials had reported the method used in the sample calculation, which may result to other biases.

Some of the limitations in the study design of included RCTs were that in the majority of analyzed studies; the reporting of the baseline characteristics data of the participants was not standardized; the inclusion and exclusion criteria were not comprehensively determined; and the age range of participants was large. Furthermore, the TCM syndrome pattern differentiation was lacking. These factors could lead to an imbalance between intervention and control groups, such as the imbalance of the types of syndrome patterns that were included, which eventually could result in reduction of the validity of outcomes, and did not reflect the uniqueness of TCM treatment based on pattern differentiation. Future investigators need to; standardize study design, standardize the reporting of baseline characteristics, and fully integrate TCM theory with their studies [184]. The duration of Diabetes (which was mainly T2DM) and DPN in the population of the selected trials was highly variable (Table3.1).The duration of diabetes in acupuncture groups ranges from 2.53±0.53 years in Wang Hui, et al 2015[168] to 12.67±1.3 in Tong Y, Guo H, Han B. 2010 [162]. However, in the control groups, the diabetes duration ranged from 2.96 ± 0.49 in Wang Hui, et al 2015[168] to 12.4±1.3 years in Tong Y., et al. 2010 [162]. Nevertheless, the DPN duration in acupuncture groups had ranged from 2.1±0.63 in trial of Tong Y., et al. 2010 [162] to 5.64± 4.77 in Jiang H, et al. 2006 [165] study (wrist ankle acu group); however, in control groups, it ranged from 1.96±0.67 years in Tong Y., et al. 2010 [162] to 5.81 ± 4.38 years in Jiang H, et al. 2006 [165]. In spite this variability in both durations of the diabetes and the DPN; however, that did not show to have any impact in the total effectiveness rates of acupuncture treatment which was very comparable in the all included studies of this review.

Further limitations of the included RCTs existed in both the study design as well as the implementation process. The methodological quality of the investigated studies was relatively poor, which itself can increase the risk of bias of the evaluation for interventions which included different acupuncture techniques.

Although in this study, 63 reports were assessed comprehensively and systematically, which are comparable to Chen Bo, et al 2012 [185] and Xiao Lu et al 2011[186] meta-analysis's reviews, only 16 RCTs were selected and the other 47 studies were excluded because they did not meet the pre-determined inclusion criteria set by this study.

An additional limitation of this meta-analysis study is including mainly English-written reports, which may has excluded some relevant and important studies written in other non-English languages such as: Japanese, Tibetan, Korean, etc. However, the studies written in the Chinese language were included also in this literature review meta-analysis after they have been carefully translated into English language using online translator tool. Nevertheless, it appears that the majority of the papers on acupuncture treatment of DPN are published mainly in English and Chinese.

The access to full text copies of most of the selected studies was challenging procedure. However, fortunately, most of the full texts of papers selected and needed for this literature review were made available. The publication time period set for the selected RCTs was 2006-2017. One trial conducted in 1998 by Abuaisha BB et al. was the only study in which the participants were followed for up to 1 year with the majority able to cease or reduce intake of pain medications post-treatment. Abuaisha and co-workers, using a 10-week course of treatment, had reported significant symptom improvement after acupuncture treatment as measured by visual analogue scores. Unfortunately, this study was not available for the assessment in this literature review, in spite of multiple full text requests which were sent to the author.

Although all the included RCTs stated the type of the randomization procedures which were used, however, only one study (Garrow AP. et al 2014 [158]) gave a full comprehensive description of the used randomization process. Another study (Tong Y. et al. 2010 [162]) gave a moderate reporting of the randomization process which had been done according to random table 2:1 and the allocations (the randomization sequences) were effectively concealed. One study (Jiang H et al. 2006 [165]) reported only that the randomization was done according to dating visit of the participants. Five studies (Lu M. et al. 2016 [159], Jin Z. et al 2011[160], Ji XQ. et al 2010 [161], Chen YL. et al 2009 [164] and FEI Ai-hua et al 2011[170]) simply mentioned that the randomization was done to distribute the participants in two groups according the random number table without any further explanation. The research design in the study by Anne Bailey et al 2017 [166] was a pragmatic effectiveness study with random allocation to either acupuncture treatment or usual care groups, with 20-25 patients per each group, according to sample size analysis. However, eventually due to multiple barriers, randomization was considered unfavorably with particular resistance to allocation to the usual care group. As a result, recruitment was eventually prioritized for the acupuncture treatment group only. The remainder 7 analyzed studies (43.75%) which are: ZHAO Hui-ling et al. 2007 [157], Zhang C. et al, 2010 [163], SUN Y-Z and XU Y-y. 2010 [167], Wang Hui et al 2015 [168], Zhao Zhixuan et al. 2010 [169], GAO Yu 2016 [171]and ZUO Lin and ZHANG Lin 2010 [172], had only mentioned that 'the patients were randomized into two groups' without any additional information. So the majority of the analyzed studies have failed to provide sufficient information to assess whether the randomization process was conducted properly or not. It was planned to evaluate the authenticity of claimed RCTs published in China [187] to drop the possibilities claimed by other meta-analysis [181] which have indicated that there was a strong possibility that some of these claimed RCTs were not real RCTs; however, the short time and resources did not permit the authenticity evaluation to be done.

Furthermore, the majority of the included studies (87.5%) did not adopt allocation concealment, which could have led to the investigators having prior knowledge of the allocation sequence, and that eventually can result in selection bias. Blinding method was reported only in two studies [158] [162] which constitute 12.5% of the tested trials. This is considered to be better than the meta-analysis of Haiyang Chen et al 2016 [188] in which Blinding data was not provided in any of its included trials. Garrow AP. et al 2014 [158] reported in the methodology section that it is designed as a single-blind, placebo-controlled RCT.

Tong Y. et al. 2010 [162] reported in full the details as to how the blinding data was carried out. The blinding procedure in the Tong Y. et al. 2010's study [162] was done by using the blinding indices, 0.32 (95% CI, 0.27 to 0.37) and −0.65 (95% CI, −0.61 to −0.69) in the acupuncture group and sham group respectively. This had indicated that 32% of patients correctly guessed the treatment identity beyond chance, while 65% of patients in the sham acupuncture group incorrectly guessed that they had received acupuncture. Nevertheless, after assessing these results, the trial investigators indicated high response bias [162], which implied that most of the study participants tend to believe that they were assigned a more effective treatment intervention.

In this literature review meta-analysis, 87.5% of the included trials did not use a blinding methodology and inferring that both the investigator and the participants knew the type of the treatment was being given. This may have introduced bias because of the confounding factor of the placebo effect. It can be observed clearly that for RCTs involving different forms of acupuncture intervention and control groups, the application of blinding to researchers and subjects would have been difficult. Nevertheless, blinding could still have been used on outcome assessors. Blinding of the outcome assessors would have been particularly significant for assessing the subjective outcome of the patients' self-reported index [188].

Participants in non-blinded RCTs would know whether they were getting real acupuncture, sham acupuncture or the vitamin control. As patients in acupuncture RCTs might have enrolled because they would have expectations for a benefit of acupuncture treatment, so they would therefore be unlikely to have strong *a priori* preferences or expectations of benefit from vitamins [181]. If participants have pre-treatment preferences for acupuncture treatment relative to the vitamin control treatment or sham control, or expectations of greater improvements from acupuncture than vitamins or other controls, these preferences and expectations may have positively biased acupuncture participants' later responses to questions about their overall total improvement [181].

Definitely, methodological research suggests that acupuncture treatment might be associated with greater outcome expectation effects compared to the standard therapies. Nevertheless, while differences in expectations may explain much of the positive benefit for the global symptom outcome, the objective outcome of the nerve conduction velocity is much less likely to be affected by participants' expectations of acupuncture benefits [181, 189]. It is unlikely that the participants' knowledge of whether they were given acupuncture or vitamins treatments would impact their nerve conduction velocity. The results of this literature review shows clearly that the total efficacy rates (table 3.2) in acupuncture treatment groups ranged from 83.33% in ZHAO Hui-ling et al. 2007 [157] to 95% in Ji XQ.et al 2010 [161] and the total efficacy rates in control groups ranged from 53.33% in ZHAO Hui-ling et al. 2007 [157] to 77.1% in ZUO Lin and ZHANG Lin 2010 [172]. The calculation of efficacy rates was based mainly on the results of NCV (SNCV and MNCV) in 93.75% of the included studies. Therefore, the uniformly positive results for the nerve conduction velocity outcomes of the majority of the analyzed RCTs are compelling even in the absence of patient blinding.

It is recommended that the blinding credibility (the masking effectiveness) has to be measured for both real acupuncture and sham acupuncture treatments [190]. In this literature review, only one study (Tong Y., et al. 2010 [162]) which constituted 6.25% of the total included studies, had assessed blinding success.

It is believed that dropout is inevitable in the course of any clinical research [181].Although most of included studies showed concordance between the number of the recruited population and the final results figures, however they failed to report clearly the withdrawal rates as well as the adverse effects. Only two studies [158, 166] which constitute 12.5% of the total tested RCTs had reported the dropout rates and reasons of those withdrawals; however, the majority (87.5%) of the included trials did not provide any specific information about drop outs. Garrow AP., et al 2014 [158], was the only study which reported in details the withdrawal from the trial. It included this information in the study design under adverse event reporting section which stated that at the beginning of each study visit, patients were asked if they had had any side effects as a result of the acupuncture treatment. Three adverse events were reported which resulted in patients withdrawing from the trial [158], two were from the acupuncture group and one from sham acupuncture group. The forms of these effects were as follows: in real acupuncture treatment group, one participant developed chest pains related to a chronic heart condition while undergoing acupuncture treatment and another patient withdrew because the participant felt that the acupuncture exacerbated her leg pain. In the sham group, one participant withdrew because she developed a localized swelling in her leg which was considered unrelated to the study. The Garrow AP., et al 2014trial [158] stated clearly that there were no cases of infections associated with the administration of acupuncture were reported.

Anne Bailey., et al 2017 [166], reported briefly that there were no adverse events from the acupuncture treatment; however, the results had shown that six participants among the 25 in the treatment group did not complete the course of acupuncture treatment. The trial [166] explained that the most prominent reason for dropping out was the concerns with other diabetes co-morbidities, as those who did not complete the treatment were more likely to have cardiovascular disease, nephropathy, peripheral vascular disease, and/or retinopathy [166].

The report of adverse events of acupuncture treatment was not adequate in the review, though the included RCTs did not have the optimal design for identifying rare but serious effects [181, 191]. Incidence rates for major adverse effects of acupuncture can be best estimated from large prospective surveys of practitioners. Four such surveys of acupuncture safety, two in Germany [192, 193] and two in the United Kingdom [194, 195], have been conducted. These confirmed that serious adverse events after acupuncture are uncommon. However, future investigators should be encouraged to monitor and report adverse events in clinical trials to evaluate the potential harms especially of the manual acupuncture treatment.

Lacking or incomplete outcome reporting might be another possible source of bias [181].

The possibility that some trials did not report these missing data could exist. However, if the missing data was not comparable between the treatment and control groups, this might result in exaggerated treatment effect of the acupuncture [196]. Furthermore, no trial reported follow-up after the treatment, therefore the acupuncture treatment long-term effect could not be established.

The type of control used in any RCT may be the major source of bias, particularly for the global improvement outcome, which would be subjective and patient-reported [181]. The analyzed studies in this review have used various types of controls that included the following; two trials (12.5%) used Sham control [162, 181], eight trials [157, 160, 161, 164, 167, 169, 170, 172] have used different forms of Methycobalamin in the control groups (oral [157, 164, 170]., intravenous [172], intramuscular [161, 167], acupoint injection [160] and one trial [169] has used intramuscular injection of both; Vit B$_1$ 100mg, VitB$_{12}$ 500µg in control group). One study [163] (6.25%) had used oral inositol in the control group, another one trial [159] (6.25%) used intravenous lipoic acid (0.6gm) and Alprastadil (10mg) in the control group and two trials [165, 171] (12.5%) used the usual western medical care in the control groups. So, most of the included trials (87.5%) had compared the acupuncture treatment versus the B vitamins, inositol, lipoic acid plus alprastadil and the usual western medicine care [165, 171]. Nevertheless, comparatively, this outcome is relatively better than that of Wei Chen, et al 2013 [181] in which no sham acupuncture was used and all included RCTs compared acupuncture versus B vitamins or no treatment.

In Jiang H, et al. 2006 [165] RCTs, treatments with specific acupuncture (wrist and ankle), was introduced as the comparator, rather than the control, for the usual acupuncture treatment. This comparator can serve as positive control so that the effectiveness of acupuncture can be measured. If the researchers choose strong positive comparator for acupuncture treatment, there would be less positive conclusions in the study [188].

In addition to the controls of sham and usual care, all the other trials in this review compared acupuncture versus B vitamins, namely, vitamin B12, B1, mecobalamin, or inositol. Although, the effectiveness of vitamin B12 on DPN has been showed by RCTs and systematic review [181, 197, 198], there was no good evidence so far to support the efficacy of mecobalamin and inositol [181, 198]. So, accordingly, these positive results of manual acupuncture should be cautiously interpreted especially when they were compared with mecobalamin or inositol.

The selection of the controls in the acupuncture RCTs is likely to have impact on the study results and conclusion. Trials using no treatment controls have the highest tendency of positive conclusions, followed by non-insertion controls, and the lowest tendency in insertion sham controls [188]. So, in order to improve the quality of the prospective acupuncture trials, the type of the control has to be carefully and appropriately chosen.

Generally, the DPN patients in the analyzed RCTs were already under treatment however they all fail to give any specific information about that treatment. Due to the significance of the pharmaceutical drugs which are mainly used for DPN treatment, especially in Europe and U.S.A, inclusion of the data of the used drugs would be an important comparison for future RCT studies. Trials duration which will reflect the acupuncture treatment duration was very variable as it ranged from minimum of 12 days (Chen YL., et al 2009 [164]) to 3 months in (Zhang C., et al, 2010 [163]).

This literature review analysis found highly diversity in the used acupuncture techniques to manage DPN in the included RCTs which specified mainly the selected acupoints and the specific manipulation used. This could be attributed mainly that in China, acupuncturists believed that treatment should be given based on individualized (tailored) syndrome pattern [181]. However, in this review, only six trials, which constitute 37.5% of the total analyzed RCTs, have provided information on patients' syndrome differentiation. So, emphasis should be paid to encourage authors to explain each syndrome differentiation ('Bianzheng' in Chinese) by using common medical terms in the future RCTs, therefore making it understandable by physicians and consumers. The diversity of manual acupuncture should also be kept in mind when interpreting the final results of any meta-analysis review.

In addition to that, with regard to acupuncture intervention, there were considerable differences in needling instruments used, number of needling sessions, selection of acupoints, depth of insertion when mentioned, method of needle manipulation, however, needle retention time was similar in the majority of the included trials and it was mainly 30 minutes. FEI Ai-hua et al 2011[170] reported retention time of 40 minutes and GAO Yu 2016 [171] of 60 minutes. Lu M. et al. 2016 [159] was the only one who failed to report the retention time.

Out of all analyzed RCTs, only Garrow AP., et al 2014 [158] trial had mentioned the practitioners'

background such as qualifications, professional affiliation, or how long they had been practicing

acupuncture in accordance with the STRICTA recommendation [155].Zhang C. et al, 2010 [163]

briefly gave information about the acupuncturist background. The majority of studies (more than

87.5%), did not provide any specific information about the practitioners' background in

compliance with STRICTA recommendations.

It is recommended that the future studies need to adopt more rigorous reporting methods of the

interventions. All the included RCTs in this review showed significant positive effects of

acupuncture treatment which in most of these RCTs was the manual acupuncture; however, no

significant difference was noticed between the use of manual acupuncture alone or in

combination with other acupuncture techniques like; EA, and moxibustion (including warm

needling). However, it was noticed clearly that not even one of the all analyzed RCTs have

reported negative outcome on using the acupuncture treatment for DPN, so, no negative study

was included. Extensive literature searches, including the excluded studies, found no published

or unpublished 'negative' studies. This might indicate obvious preferential publication of positive

studies might be due to the rejection of journal editors to negative trials, the lack of awareness to

register clinical trials in China, or the inaccessibility to unpublished data [25]. The extensive

systemic research search undertaken has shown that several initiatives are underway with the

objective to guarantee that all trials, both positive and negative, will be published in the future.

These include efforts to promote the prospective registration of all clinical trials, publication of

clinical trial protocols, and reporting of negative clinical trials [181].

In comparison to other similar reviews, one of unique features of this study is that its results are

based mainly on the novel STRICTA-P tool which has been used for the first time in this

literature review analysis. In general, articles of acupuncture treatment are more likely to provide

detailed information on acupoints and needling manipulation because these are what the

acupuncturist readers are interested in [25]. While our assessment tool was the newly introduced

STRICTA-P tool, Wei Chen et al 2013 [181] assessment was based on CONSORT that were in accordance with Chen Bo's study [185], which implied attention should also be paid to methodological issues for the future clinical investigator. The CONSORT Statement[155] comprises a 25-item checklist and a flow diagram is considered to be a general , not specific, quality assessment tool which can be applied on all random controlled trials, however the new STRICTA-P quality assessment tool which has been proposed through this literature review study, includes a 22-item which in addition to focusing on the specific acupuncture intervention procedures, Acupuncture rationale, Details of needling, Treatment regimen, Other components of treatment, Practitioner background and Control or comparator interventions acupuncturist and control groups, it also focuses on; Randomization, blinding process and dropouts (withdrawals). So, for acupuncture RCTs, it would be more specific, credible and statistically powerful to apply STRICTA-P tool rather than CONSORT statement.

Compared to similar reviews, for example; Chen Bo's study [185], has included RCTs which were lacking the details of needling, details of other intervention, practitioner background and so on; however, in this meta-analysis review, the reports on details of needling were satisfactory. This difference might be explained by the different inclusion criteria. This meta-analysis review included RCTs that used different acupuncture techniques (manual acupuncture, EA, warm acupuncture, scalp acupuncture, wrist and ankle acupuncture).Similarly, the Chen Bo's study [185], included all types of acupuncture (manual acupuncture, acupoint injection, scalp acupuncture, etc). However, Wei Chen et al 2013[181] review included manual acupuncture only. Furthermore, this meta-analysis used stricter inclusion criteria than Chen Bo's study [185], but comparable to Wei Chen et al 2013 [181], therefore, we included fewer RCTs than Chen Bo's study [185].

## 5.0 Conclusion

This literature review aimed to explore, the effectiveness and safety of the use of acupuncture treatment in the management of DPN as add-on complementary therapy. In fact, the uniform consistent results of the total efficacy rates based on nerve velocity studies before and after acupuncture treatment in the majority of the included RCTs support this notion. However, the heterogeneity of the included trials did not allow us making a firm conclusion on the effectiveness of acupuncture treatment, and what is most effective acupuncture treatment protocol to follow. Since the same treatment rational was rarely used in different studies, it is difficult to compare results. The robustness of the results of the included trials could not be determined due to the fact that the majority of the included trials were of 'inadequate methodology' and low study population with multiple methodological and reporting biases. So, the reported beneficial effect of the acupuncture treatment for DPN cannot be taken as confirmative conclusion. Nevertheless, to ensure evidence-based clinical practice, further rigorous placebo-controlled, randomized trials are critically needed. For these prospective trials, more attention would be definitely needed to reduce the multiple risks of bias, and the reporting quality must be improved by complying with the CONSORT, STRICTA statements and possible application of the new quality assessment tool used in this study (STRICTA-P) as well as adequate and proper training of the acupuncture treatment researchers about all these issues aiming to get robust highly reliable prospective RCTs with much less bias.

## 6.0 Future Perspectives

➤ Great emphasis should be paid to encourage authors to explain each syndrome differentiation ('Bianzheng' in Chinese) by using common medical terms, therefore making it understandable and ensuring uniqueness of traditional Chinese medicine in tailoring the acupuncture treatment for DPN.

➤ Including higher number of study participants to increase the power and strengthen the robustness of these prospective studies. Furthermore, sample calculation method need to be performed and well reported to minimize the related bias.

➤ Investigators ought to standardize study design, the used diagnosis criteria, the reporting of baseline characteristics, and fully integrate TCM theory in their studies.

➤ Randomization and blinding methodology need to be well reported in the study design protocol and also well implicated throughout the trial. Furthermore, it is recommended that the blinding credibility (the masking effectiveness) has to be measured for both real acupuncture and sham acupuncture treatments.

➤ Investigators and acupuncturists need to be encouraged to monitor and report meticulously the dropouts and the adverse events in acupuncture clinical trials to evaluate the potential harms in general and especially of the manual acupuncture treatment.

➤ Encouraging the use and proper reporting of the Intention to treat (ITT) analysis of all prospective acupuncture RCTs. This ITT analysis means that all patients who will be enrolled and randomly allocated to acupuncture treatment are included in the analysis and are analyzed in the groups to which they are randomized.

➤ Emphasis needs to be paid on the inclusion of the long term follow up of the participants in such prospective trials for example once or twice annually. This long term follow up protocol would help to assess the sustainability of acupuncture treatment for DPN.

➤ Since the selection of the type of control used in acupuncture RCTs is thought to be a major source of bias and in order to improve the quality of prospective acupuncture RCTs, the control is to be carefully chosen. It is highly recommended to select the sham acupuncture control because it carries the least risk of bias in acupuncture intervention trials.

➤ Continuous regular intense promotion of the academic discussion between several acupuncture and TCM research groups in China and internationally aiming to achieve some forms of consensuses about the possible standardized acupuncture treatment protocols as well as considering the tailoring process according the syndrome differentiation of the participants. So, future RCTs ought to adopt more rigorous reporting of interventions and standardized acupuncture protocol to enhance the robustness, comparability and the replication of acupuncture prospective RCTs.

➢ Implementing measures which can cancel or highly reduce the possible current publication bias of acupuncture RCTs and enhancing all the initiatives which aim to guarantee that all trials, both positive and negative, will be published in the future. These would include the initiatives to promote and well observe the prospective registration of all the clinical RCTs, publication of acupuncture clinical RCTs' protocols, and adequately reporting of negative clinical trials.

# REFERENCES

## References

1. http://www.idf.org/membership/eur/malta (Accessed last on 3-07-2017)

2. Kumar S, Ashe HC, Parnell LN, Fernando DJS, Tsigos C, Young RJ, Ward JD, Boulton AJM: The prevalence of foot ulceration and its correlates in type 2 diabetes: a population-based study. Diabetic Med11: 480-484, 1994.

3. Cabezas-Cerrato J: The prevalence of diabetic neuropathy in Spain: a study in primary care and hospital clinic groups. Diabetologia41: 1263-1269, 1998.

4. Boulton AJM, Malik RA, Arezzo JC, Sosenko JM: Diabetic somatic neuropathies: a technical review.Diabetes Care 27:1458 -1486, 2004.

5. Boulton AJM, Gries FA, Jervell JA: Guidelines for the diagnosis and outpatient management of diabetic peripheral neuropathy. Diabetic Med15: 508-514, 1998.

6. Yagihashi S, Mizukami H, Sugimoto K: Mechanism of diabetic neuropathy: Where are we now and where to go? J Diabetes Investig. 2011, 2: 18-32

7. Kihara M, Weerasuriya A, Low PA. Endoneurial blood flow in rat sciatic nerve during development. J Physiol 1991; 439: 351–360.

8. Sugimoto H, Monafo WW. Regional blood flow in sciatic nerve, biceps femoris muscle, and truncal skin in response to hemorrhagic hypotension. J Trauma 1987; 27: 1025– 1030.

9. Smith DR, Kobrine AI, Rizzoli HV. Absence of autoregulation in peripheral nerve blood flow. J Neurol Sci 1977; 33: 347– 352.

10. Sima AA, Nathaniel V, Prashar A, et al. Endoneurial microvessels in human diabetic neuropathy. Endothelial cell dysjunction and lack of treatment effect by aldose reductase inhibitor. Diabetes 1991; 40: 1090–1099.

11. Grover-Johnson NM, Baumann FG, Imparato AM, et al. Abnormal innervation of lower limb epineurial arterioles inhuman diabetes. Diabetologia 1981; 20: 31–38.

# References

12. Beggs J, Johnson PC, Olafsen A, et al. Innervation of the vasa nervorum: changes in human diabetics. J Neuropathol Exp Neurol 1992; 51: 612–629.

13. KE. Epidemiology and impact on quality of life of post herpetic neuralgia and painful diabetic neuropathy. Clin J Pain2002; 18:350−4.

14. Ziegler D, Sohr CGH, Nourooz-Zadeh J. Oxidative stress and antioxidant defense in relation to the severity of diabetic polyneuropathy and cardiovascular autonomic neuropathy. Diabetes Care2004;27:2178−83.

15. Yagihashi S, Matsunaga M. Ultra structural pathology of peripheral nerves in patients with diabetic neuropathy.Tohoku J Exp Med 1979; 129: 357–366.

16. Dyck PJ, Giannini C. Pathologic alterations in the diabetic neuropathies of humans: a review. J Neuropathol Exp Neurol 1996; 55: 1181–1193.

17. Dyck PJ, Karnes J, O'Brien P, et al. Spatial pattern of nerve fiber abnormality indicative of pathologic mechanism. Am JPathol 1984; 117: 225–238.

18. Dyck PJ, Karnes JL, O'Brien P, et al. The spatial distribution of fiber loss in diabetic polyneuropathy suggests ischemia. Ann Neurol 1986; 19: 440–449.

19. Llewelyn JG, Thomas PK, Gilbey SG, et al. Pattern of myelinated fibre loss in the sural nerve in neuropathy related to type 1 (Insulin-dependent) diabetes. Diabetologia 1988; 31: 162–167.

20. Thrainsdottir S, Malik RA, Dahlin LB, et al. Endoneurial capillary abnormalities presage deterioration of glucose tolerance and accompany peripheral neuropathy in man. Diabetes 2003; 52: 2615–2622.

21. Malik RA, Tesfaye S, Newrick PG, et al. Sural nerve pathology in diabetic patients with minimal but progressive neuropathy. Diabetologia 2005; 48: 578–585.

22. McCarthy BG, Hsieh ST, Stocks A, et al. Cutaneous innervations in sensory neuropathies: evaluation by skin biopsy. Neurology 1995; 45: 1848–1855.

23. Kennedy WR, Wendelschafer-Crabb G, Johnson T. Quantitation of epidermal nerves

References

24. Polydefkis M, Hauer P, Sheth S, et al. The time course of epidermal nerve fibre regeneration: studies in normal controls and in people with diabetes, with and without neuropathy. Brain 2004; 127: 1606–1615.

25. Shun CT, Chang YC, Wu HP, et al. Skin denervation in type 2diabetes: correlations with diabetic duration and functional impairments. Brain 2004; 127: 1593–1605.

26. Malik RA, Kallinikos P, Abbott CA, et al. Corneal confocal microscopy: a non-invasive surrogate of nerve fibre damage and repair in diabetic patients. Diabetologia 2003; 46: 683–638.

27. Hossain P, Sachdev A, Malik RA. Early detection of diabetic peripheral neuropathy with corneal confocal microscopy. Lancet 2005; 366: 1340–1343.

28. Quattrini C, Tavakoli M, Jeziorska M, et al. Surrogate markers of small fiber damage in human diabetic neuropathy.Diabetes 2007; 56: 2148–2154.

29. Mehra S, Tavakoli M, Kallinikos PA, et al. Corneal confocal microscopy detects early nerve regeneration after pancreas transplantation in patients with type 1 diabetes. Diabetes Care 2007; 30: 2608–2612.

30. Green AQ, Krishnan S, Finucane FM, Rayman G: Altered C-fiber function as an indicator of early peripheral neuropathy in individuals with impaired glucose tolerance. Diabetes care. 2010, 33: 174-176.

31. Khan GM, Chen SR, Pan HL: Role of primary afferent nerves in allodynia caused by diabetic neuropathy in rats. Neuroscience. 2002, 114: 291-299.

32. Cheliout-Heraut F, Zrek N, Khemliche H, Varnet O, Seret-Begue D, Martinez M, Nizou R, Bour F: Exploration of small fibers for testing diabetic neuropathies. Joint Bone Spine. 2005, 72: 412-415.

References

33. Goto Y, Hotta N, Shigeta Y, et al. Effects of an aldose reductase inhibitor, epalrestat, on diabetic neuropathy. Clinical benefit and indication for the drug assessed from the results of a placebo-controlled double-blind study. Biomed Pharmacother 1995; 49: 269–277.

34. Hotta N, Akanuma Y, Kawamori R, et al. Long-term clinical effects of epalrestat, an aldose reductase inhibitor, on diabetic peripheral neuropathy: the 3-year, multicenter, comparative Aldose Reductase Inhibitor-Diabetes Complications Trial. Diabetes Care 2006; 29: 1538–1544.

35. Hotta N, Kawamori R, Atsumi Y, et al. Stratified analyses for selecting appropriate target patients with diabetic peripheral neuropathy for long-term treatment with an aldosereductase inhibitor, epalrestat. Diabet Med 2008; 25: 818–825.

36. Pfeifer MA, Schumer MP, Gelber DA. Aldose reductase inhibitors: the end of an era or the need for different trial designs? Diabetes 1997; 46(Suppl 2): S82–S89.

37. Ryan GJ. New pharmacologic approaches to treating diabetic retinopathy. Am J Health Syst Pharm 2007; 17(Suppl 12):S15–S21.

38. Gabbay KH. Hyperglycemia, polyol metabolism, and complications of diabetes mellitus. Annu Rev Med 1975; 26: 521–536.

39. Kinoshita JH. A thirty-year journey in the polyol pathway. Exp Eye Res 1990; 50: 567–573.

40. Jakobsen J, Sidenius P. Nerve morphology in experimental diabetes. Clin Physiol 1985; 5(Suppl 5): 9–13.

41. Greene DA, Lattimer SA, Sima AA. Sorbitol, phosphoinositides, and sodium-potassium-ATPase in the pathogenesisof diabetic complications. N Engl J Med 1987; 316: 599–606.

42. Greene DA, Sima AA, Stevens MJ, et al. Complications: neuropathy, pathogenetic considerations. Diabetes Care1992; 15: 1902–1925.

43. Dyck PJ, Sherman WR, Hallcher LM, et al. Human diabetic endoneurial sorbitol, fructose, and myo-inositol related to sural nerve morphometry. Ann Neurol 1980; 8: 590–596.

95

# References

44. Dyck PJ, Zimmerman BR, Vilen TH, et al. Nerve glucose,fructose, sorbitol, myo-inositol, and fiber degeneration and regeneration in diabetic neuropathy. N Engl J Med 1988;319: 542–548.

45. Drel VR, Mashtalir N, Ilnytska O, et al. The leptin-deficient (ob/ob) mouse: a new animal model of peripheral neuropathy of type 2 diabetes and obesity. Diabetes 2006; 55:3335–3343.

46. Obrosova IG, Ilnytska O, Lyzogubov VV, et al. High-fat diet induced neuropathy of pre-diabetes and obesity: effects of "healthy" diet and aldose reductase inhibition. Diabetes2007; 56: 2598–2608.

47. Yagihashi S, Yamagishi S, Wada R, et al. Galactosemic neuropathy in transgenic mice for human aldose reductase. Diabetes 1996; 45: 56–59.

48. Yagihashi S, Yamagishi SI, Wada R, et al. Neuropathy in diabetic mice over expressing human aldose reductase and effects of aldose reductase inhibitor. Brain 2001; 124: 2448–2458.

49. Uehara K, Yamagishi S, Otsuki S, et al. Effects of polyol pathway hyperactivity on protein kinase C activity, nociceptive peptide expression, and neuronal structure in dorsal root ganglia in diabetic mice. Diabetes 2004; 53:3239–3247.

50. Ho EC, Lam KS, Chen YS, et al. Aldose reductase-deficient mice are protected from delayed motor nerve conduction velocity, increased c-Jun NH2-terminal kinase activation, depletion of reduced glutathione, increased superoxide accumulation, and DNA damage. Diabetes 2006; 55: 1946–1953.

51. Yagihashi S, Yamagishi SI, Mizukami H, et al. Escape phenomenon from polyol pathway to other metabolic cascades may underlie nerve conduction delay in severely hyperglycemic AR-deficient mice. 68th American Diabetes Association, San Francisco, USA, June 6–10, 2008

52. Hwang YC, Shaw S, Kaneko M, et al. Aldose reductase pathway mediates JAK-STAT signaling: a novel axis in myocardial ischemic injury. FASEB J 2005; 19: 795–797.

# References

53. Iwata K, Matsuno K, Nishinaka T, et al. Aldose reductase inhibitors improve myocardial reperfusion injury in mice bya dual mechanism. J Pharmacol Sci 2006; 102: 37–46.

54. Cheung AK, Lo AC, So KF, et al. Gene deletion and pharmacological inhibition of aldose reductase protect against retinal ischemic injury. Exp Eye Res 2007; 85: 608–616.

55. Yeung CM, Lo AC, Cheung AK, et al. More severe type 2diabetes-associated ischemic stroke injury is alleviated in aldose reductase-deficient mice. J Neurosci Res 2010; 88:2026–2034.

56. Agardh CD, Agardh E, Obrosova IG, et al. The aldose reductase inhibitor fidarestat suppresses ischemia-reperfusion induced inflammatory response in rat retina. Pharmacology2009; 84: 257–263.

57. Yagihashi S, Mizukami H, Ogasawara S, et al. The role of the polyol pathway in acute kidney injury caused by hind limb ischaemia in mice. J Pathol 2010; 220: 530–541.

58. Obrosova IG, Maksimchyk Y, Pacher P, et al. Evaluation ofthe aldose reductase inhibitor fidarestat on ischemia reperfusion injury in rat retina. Int J Mol Med 2010; 26: 135–142.

59. Nukada H, Lynch CD, McMorran PD. Aggravated reperfusion injury in STZ-diabetic nerve. J Peripher Nerv Syst 2002;7: 37–43.

60. Baba M, Nukada H, McMorran D, et al. Prolonged ischemic conduction failure after reperfusion in diabetic nerve. Muscle Nerve 2006; 33: 350–355.

61. Kasajima H, Yamagishi S, Sugai S, et al. Enhanced in situ expression of aldose reductase in peripheral nerve andrenal glomeruli in diabetic patients. Virchows Arch 2001;439: 46–54.

62. Yamagishi S, Uehara K, Otsuki S, et al. Differential influenceof increased polyol pathway on protein kinase C expressions between endoneurial and epineurial tissues in diabeticmice. J Neurochem 2003; 87: 497–507.

63. Yagihashi S. The pathogenesis of diabetic neuropathy. Diabetes Metab Res Rev 1995; 11: 193–225.

References

64. Thornalley PJ. Glycation in diabetic neuropathy: characteristics, consequences, causes, and therapeutic options. Int Rev Neurobiol 2002; 50: 37–57.

65. Sugimoto K, Yasujima M, Yagihashi S. Role of advanced glycation end products in diabetic neuropathy. Curr PharmDes 2008; 14: 953–961.

66. Sugimoto K, Nishizawa Y, Horiuchi S, et al. Localization inhuman diabetic peripheral nerve of N(epsilon)-carboxymethyllysine-protein adducts, an advanced glycation end product. Diabetologia 1997; 40: 1380–1387.

67. Sekido H, Suzuki T, Jomori T, et al. Reduced cell replication and induction of apoptosis by advanced glycation end products in rat Schwann cells. Biochem Biophys Res Commun2004; 320: 241–248.

68. Ryle C, Leow CK, Donaghy M. Non enzymatic glycation of peripheral and central nervous system proteins in experimental diabetes mellitus. Muscle Nerve 1997; 20: 577–584.

69. Duran-Jimenez B, Dobler D, Moffatt S, et al. Advanced glycation end products in extracellular matrix proteins contribute to the failure of sensory nerve regeneration in diabetes. Diabetes 2009; 58: 2893–2903.

70. Wada R, Yagihashi S. Role of advanced glycation end products and their receptors in development of diabetic neuropathy. Ann N Y Acad Sci 2005; 1043: 598–604.

71. Toth C, Rong LL, Yang C, et al. Receptor for advanced glycation end products (RAGEs) and experimental diabetic neuropathy. Diabetes 2008; 57: 1002–1017.

72. Kihara M, Schmelzer JD, Poduslo JF, et al. Aminoguanidine effects on nerve blood flow, vascular permeability, electrophysiology, and oxygen free radicals. Proc Natl Acad Sci USA1991; 88: 6107–6111.

73. Yagihashi S, Kamijo M, Baba M, et al. Effect of aminoguanidine on functional and structural abnormalities in peripheral nerve of STZ-induced diabetic rats. Diabetes 1992; 41: 47–52.

# References

74. Wada R, Nishizawa Y, Yagihashi N, et al. Effects of OPB-9195, anti-glycation agent, on experimental diabetic neuropathy. Eur J Clin Invest 2001; 31: 513–520.

75. Cameron NE, Gibson TM, Nangle MR, et al. Inhibitors of advanced glycation end product formation and neurovascular dysfunction in experimental diabetes. Ann N Y AcadSci 2005; 1043: 784–792.

76. Nishizawa Y, Wada R, Baba M, et al. Neuropathy induced by exogenously administered advanced glycation end-products.J Diabetes Invest 2010; 1: 40–49.

77. Haupt E, Ledermann H, Ko"pckeW. Benfotiamine in the treatment of diabetic polyneuropathy – a three-week randomized, controlled pilot study (BEDIP study). Int J ClinPharmacol Ther 2005; 43: 71–77.98.

78. Greene DA, Stevens MJ, Obrosova I, et al. Glucose-induced oxidative stress and programmed cell death in diabetic neuropathy. Eur J Pharmacol 1999; 375: 217–223.

79. Pop-Busui R, Sima A, Stevens M. Diabetic neuropathy and oxidative stress. Diabetes Metab Res Rev 2006; 22: 257–273.

80. Obrosova IG. Diabetes and the peripheral nerve. Biochim Biophys Acta 2009; 1792: 931–940.

81. Cameron NE, Cotter MA. Potential therapeutic approaches to the treatment or prevention of diabetic neuropathy: evidence from experimental studies. Diabet Med 1993; 10:593–605.

82. Cameron NE, Cotter MA, Maxfield EK. Anti-oxidant treatment prevents the development of peripheral nerve dysfunctionin streptozotocin-diabetic rats. Diabetologia 1993;36: 299–304.

83. Kishi Y, Schmelzer JD, Yao JK, et al. Alpha-lipoic acid: effect on glucose uptake, sorbitol pathway, and energy metabolism in experimental diabetic neuropathy. Diabetes 1999; 48:2045–2051.

# References

84. Stevens MJ, Obrosova I, Cao X, et al. Effects of DL-alpha lipoic acid on peripheral nerve conduction, blood flow, energy metabolism, and oxidative stress in experimental diabetic neuropathy. Diabetes 2000; 49: 1006–1015.

85. Drel VR, Pacher P, Stevens MJ, et al. Aldose reductase inhibition counteracts nitrosative stress and poly(ADP-ribose)polymerase activation in diabetic rat kidney and high glucose-exposed human mesangial cells. Free Radic BiolMed 2006; 40: 1454–1465.

86. Obrosova IG, Van Huysen C, Fathallah L, et al. An aldose reductase inhibitor reverses early diabetes-induced changes in peripheral nerve function, metabolism, and anti-oxidative defense. FASEB J 2002; 16: 123–125.

87. Ziegler D, Hanefeld M, Ruhnau KJ, et al. Treatment of symptomatic diabetic peripheral neuropathy with the antioxidant alpha-lipoic acid. A 3-week multicentre randomized controlled trial (ALADIN Study). Diabetologia 1995; 38:1425–1433.

88. Way KJ, Katai N, King GL. Protein kinase C and the development of diabetic vascular complications. Diabet Med 2001;18: 945–959.

89. Geraldes P, King GL. Activation of protein kinase C isoforms and its impact on diabetic complications. Circ Res 2010;106: 1319–1331.

90. Nakamura J, Kato K, Hamada Y, et al. A protein kinase C-beta-selective inhibitor ameliorates neural dysfunction in streptozotocin-induced diabetic rats. Diabetes 1999; 48:2090–2095.

91. Kamiya H, Nakamura J, Hamada Y, et al. Polyol pathway and protein kinase C activity of rat Schwannoma cells. Diabetes Metab Res Rev 2003; 19: 131–139.

92. Cameron NE, Cotter MA. Effects of protein kinase Cbeta inhibition on neurovascular dysfunction in diabetic rats: interaction with oxidative stress and essential fatty acid dysmetabolism. Diabetes Metab Res Rev 2002; 18: 315–323.

93. Sasase T, Yamada H, Sakoda K, et al. Novel protein kinase C-beta isoform selective inhibitor JTT-010 ameliorates both hyper- and hypoalgesia in streptozotocin- induced diabetic rats. Diabetes Obes Metab 2005; 7: 586–594.

94. Casellini CM, Barlow PM, Rice AL, et al. A 6-month, randomized, double-masked, placebo-controlled study evaluating the effects of the protein kinase C-beta inhibitor ruboxistaurin on skin microvascular blood flow and other measures of diabetic peripheral neuropathy. Diabetes Care 2007; 30:896–902.

95. Shangguan Y, Hall KE, Neubig RR, et al. Diabetic neuropathy: inhibitory G protein dysfunction involves PKC-dependent phosphorylation of Goalpha. J Neurochem 2003; 86:1006–1014.

96. Sakaue Y, Sanada M, Sasaki T, et al. Amelioration of retarded neurite outgrowth of dorsal root ganglion neurons by over expression of PKC delta in diabetic rats. Neuro report 2003;14: 431–436.

97. Younger DS, Rosoklija G, Hays AP, et al. Diabetic peripheral neuropathy: a clinic pathologic and immune histochemical analysis of sural nerve biopsies. Muscle Nerve 1996; 19: 722–727.

98. Satoh J, Yagihashi S, Toyota T. The possible role of tumor necrosis factor-alpha in diabetic polyneuropathy. Exp Diabesity Res 2003; 4: 65–71.

99. Pop-Busui R, Marinescu V, Van Huysen C, et al. Dissection of metabolic, vascular, and nerve conduction interrelationships in experimental diabetic neuropathy by cyclooxygenase inhibition and acetyl-L-carnitine administration. Diabetes2002; 51: 2619–2628.

100. Kellogg AP, Converso K, Wiggin T, et al. Effects of cyclooxygenase-2 gene inactivation on cardiac autonomic and left ventricular function in experimental diabetes. Am J Physiol Heart Circ Physiol 2009; 296: H453–H461.

101. Yamagishi S, Ogasawara S, Mizukami H, et al. Correction of protein kinase C activity and macrophage migration in peripheral nerve by pioglitazone, peroxisome proliferator activated-gamma-ligand, in insulin-deficient diabetic rats.J Neurochem 2008; 104: 491–499.

102. Tomlinson DR. Mitogen-activated protein kinases as glucose transducers for diabetic complications. Diabetologia 1999; 42: 1271–1281.

# References

103. Du Y, Tang J, Li G, et al. Effects of p38 MAPK inhibition on early stages of diabetic retinopathy and sensory nerve function. Invest Ophthalmol Vis Sci 2010; 51: 2158–2164.

104. Towns R, Pietropaolo M, Wiley JW. Stimulation of autophagy by autoantibody-mediated activation of death receptor cascades. Autophagy 2008; 4: 715–716.

105. Ramos KM, Jiang Y, Svensson CI, et al. Pathogenesis of spinally mediated hyperalgesia in diabetes. Diabetes 2007; 56:1569–1576.

106. Doupis J, Lyons TE, Wu S, et al. Microvascular reactivity and inflammatory cytokines in painful and painless peripheral diabetic neuropathy. J Clin Endocrinol Metab 2009; 94:2157–2163.

107. Saini AK, Kumar HSA, Sharma SS. Preventive and curative effect of edaravone on nerve functions and oxidative stress in experimental diabetic neuropathy. Eur J Pharmacol 2007; 568: 164–172.

108. Tomlinson DR, Fernyhough P, Diemel LT. Role of neurotrophins in diabetic neuropathy and treatment with nerve growth factors. Diabetes 1997; 46(Suppl 2): S43–S49.

109. Zochodne DW. Neurotrophins and other growth factors in diabetic neuropathy. Semin Neurol 1996; 16: 153–161.

110. Apfel SC. Neurotrophic factors in the therapy of diabetic neuropathy. Am J Med 1999; 107: 34S–42S.

111. Pittenger G, Vinik A. Nerve growth factor and diabetic neuropathy. Exp Diabesity Res 2003; 4: 271–285.

112. Hellweg R, Hartung HD. Endogenous levels of nerve growth factor (NGF) are altered in experimental diabetes mellitus: a possible role for NGF in the pathogenesis of diabetic neuropathy. J Neurosci Res 1990; 26: 258–267.

113. Anand P, Terenghi G, Warner G, et al. The role of endogenous nerve growth factor in human diabetic neuropathy. Nat Med 1996; 2: 703–707.

# References

114. Apfel SC, Kessler JA, Adornato BT, et al. Recombinant human nerve growth factor in the treatment of diabetic polyneuropathy. NGF Study Group. Neurology 1998; 51: 695–702.

115. Murakami T, Arai M, Sunada Y, et al. VEGF 164 gene transfer by electroporation improves diabetic sensory neuropathy in mice. J Gene Med 2006; 8: 773–781.

116. Terashima T, Kojima H, Fujimiya M, et al. The fusion of bone-marrow-derived proinsulin-expressing cells with nerve cells underlies diabetic neuropathy. Proc Natl Acad Sci USA 2005; 102: 12525–12530.

117. Busik JV, Tikhonenko M, Bhatwadekar A, et al. Diabetic neuropathy is associated with bone marrow neuropathy and a depressed peripheral clock. J Exp Med 2010; 206: 2897–2906.

118. Imai J, Katagiri H, Yamada T, et al. Regulation of pancreatic beta cell mass by neuronal signals from the liver. Science 2008; 322: 1250–1254.

119. James Lausier, William C. Diaz, Violet Roskens, et al. Vagal control of pancreatic β-cell proliferation. Am J Physiol Endocrinol Metab. 2010 Nov; 299(5): E786–E793.

120. KE. Epidemiology and impact on quality of life of post herpetic neuralgia and painful diabetic neuropathy. Clin J Pain2002;18:350−4.

121. DyckPJ, Katz KM, Karnes JL, Litchy WJ, Klein R, Pach JM: The prevalence by staged severity of various types of diabetic neuropathy, retinopathy and nephropathy in a population-based cohort: The Rochester Diabetic Neuropathy study. Neurology 43:817 - 824, 1993.

122. Hurtak JJ. An overview of acupuncture medicine. JAltern Complement Med2002; 8:535−8.

123. Dyck PJ, Albers JW, Andersen H, et al; Toronto Expert Panel on Diabetic Neuropathy. Diabetic polyneuropathies: update on research definition, diagnostic criteria and estimation of severity. Diabetes Metab Res Rev 2011;27(7):620–628.

# References

124. England JD, Gronseth GS, Franklin G, et al; American Academy of Neurology; American Association of Electrodiagnostic Medicine; American Academy of Physical Medicine and Rehabilitation. Distal symmetric polyneuropathy: a definition for clinical research: report of the American Academy of Neurology, the American Association of Electrodiagnostic Medicine, and the American Academy of Physical Medicine and Rehabilitation. Neurology 2005;64(2):199–207.

125. Perkins BA, Bril V. Electrophysiologic testing in diabetic neuropathy. In: Zochodne DW, Malik RA, eds. Handbook of Clinical Neurology, Vol. 126 (3rd Series) Diabetes and the Nervous System. Amsterdam, The Netherlands: Elsevier BV; 2014:235–248.

126. Perkins BA, Ngo M, Bril V. Symmetry of nerve conduction studies in different stages of diabetic polyneuropathy. Muscle Nerve 2002; 25(2):212–217.

127. Abbott CA, Carrington AL, Ashe H, Every L, Whalley A, Van Ross ERE, Boulton AJM: The North-West Diabetes Foot Care Study: incidence of, and risk factors for new diabetic foot ulceration in a community-based patient cohort. Diabetic Med 2002; **19**:377 -384.

128. Mayfield JA, Sugarman JR: The use of Semmes-Weinstein monofilament and other threshold tests for preventing foot ulceration and amputation in people with diabetes. J Fam Pract 2000; 49 (Suppl.):517-529.

129. Mendell JR, Sahenk Z: Painful sensory neuropathy. N Engl J Med 2003; **348**: 1243-1255.

130. Ulugol A, Karadag HC, Tamer M: Involvement of adenosine in the anti-allodynic effect of amitriptyline in streptozotocin-induced diabetic rats. Neurosci Lett 2002; 328:129 -132.

131. Harati Y, Gooch C, Swenson M, Edelman S, Greene D, Raskin P, Donofrio P, Cornblath D: Double-blind randomized trial of tramadol for the treatment of the pain of diabetic neuropathy. Neurology1998; **50**: 1841-1846.

132. Feldman EL, Stevens MJ, Thomas PK, Brown MB, Canal N, Greene DA: A practical two-step quantitative clinical and electrophysiological assessment for the diagnosis and staging of diabetic neuropathy. Diabetes Care1996; **17**: 1281-1289.

References

133. Argoff CE, Backonja MM, Belgrade MJ, Bennett GJ, Clark MR, Cole BE, Fishbain DA, Irving GA, McCarberg BH, McLean MJ: Consensus guidelines: treatment planning and options. Diabetic peripheral neuropathic pain. Mayo Clin Proc. 2006, 81 (Suppl 4): S12-S25.

134. Gillespie EA, Gillespie BW, Stevens MJ: Painful diabetic neuropathy: impact of an alternative approach. Diabetes care. 2007, 30: 999-1001.

135. Abuaisha BB, Costanzi JB, Boulton AJ: Acupuncture for the treatment of chronic painful peripheral diabetic neuropathy: a long-term study. Diabetes Res Clin Pract. 1998, 39: 115-121.

136. Lao L: Traditional Chinese Medicine. In Essentials of Complementary and Alternative Medicine. Jonas WB, Levin JS, Eds. Baltimore, Md., Lippincott Williams and Wilkins, 1999, p. 216–232

137. Maggie B. Covington. Traditional Chinese Medicine in the Treatment of Diabetes. Diabetes Spectrum 2001 Aug; 14(3): 154-159.

138. Kaptchuk TJ: The Web That Has No Weaver: Understanding Chinese Medicine. Chicago, Congdon & Weed, 1983

139. Parker MJ: Traditional Chinese Medicine. In Clinician's Complete Reference to Complementary & Alternative Medicine. Novey DW, Ed. St. Louis, Mo., Mosby, 2000, p. 203–218

140. Chen DC, Gong DQ, Zhai Y: Diabetes acupuncture research. J Trad Chinese Med 1994; 14:163–166.

141. Mao-liang Q: The treatment of diabetes by acupuncture. J Chinese Med 1984; 15:3–5.

142. Helms JM: Acupuncture Energetics: A Clinical Approach for Physicians. Berkeley, Calif., Medical Acupuncture, 1995

143. Ziegler D, Sohr CGH, Nourooz-Zadeh J. Oxidative stress and antioxidant defense in relation to the severity of diabetic polyneuropathy and cardiovascular autonomic neuropathy. Diabetes Care2004; 27:2178−83.

# References

144. Goldman N, Chen M, Fujita T, Xu Q, Peng W, Liu W, Jensen TK, Pei Y, Wang F, Han X: Adenosine A1 receptors mediate local anti-nociceptive effects of acupuncture. Nat Neurosci. 2010, 13: 883-888.

145. White A, Cummings TM, Filshie J: An Introduction to Western Medical Acupuncture. 2008, Edinburgh: Churchill Livingstone/Elsevier

146. Han JS: Acupuncture and endorphins. Neurosci Lett. 2004, 361: 258-261.

147. Vickers AJ, Cronin AM, Maschino AC, Lewith G, MacPherson H, Foster NE, Sherman KJ, Witt CM, Linde K, Acupuncture Trialists C: Acupuncture for chronic pain: individual patient data meta-analysis. Arch Intern Med. 2012, 172: 1444-145

148. Lawrence Leung. Neurophysiological Basis of Acupuncture-induced Analgesia. An Updated Review. J Acupunct Meridian Stud 2012; 5(6):261e270

149. Zhou Y, Sun YH, Shen JM, Han JS. Increased release of immune reactive CCK-8 by electroacupuncture and enhancement of electroacupuncture analgesia by CCK-B antagonist in rat spinal cord. Neuropeptides. 1993; 24:139e144.

150. Han JS, Ding XZ, Fan SG. Cholecystokinin octapeptide (CCK-8):antagonism to electroacupuncture analgesia and a possible role in electroacupuncture tolerance. Pain. 1986; 27:101e115.

151. Huang C, Hu ZP, Jiang SZ, Li HT, Han JS, Wan Y. CCK(B) receptor antagonist L365, 260 potentiates the efficacy to and reverses chronic tolerance to electroacupuncture-induced analgesia in mice. Brain Res Bull. 2007; 71:447e451.

152. Chen XH, Geller EB, Adler MW. CCK(B) receptors in the periaqueductal grey are involved in electroacupuncture antinociception in the rat cold water tail-flick test. Neuropharmacology. 1998; 37:751e757.

153. Lee G, Rho S, Shin M, Hong M, Min B, Bae H. The association of cholecystokinin-A receptor expression with the responsiveness of electroacupuncture analgesic effects in rat. Neuroscience Lett. 2002; 325:17e20.

References

154. World Health Organization. Definition, Diagnosis and Classification of Diabetes mellitus and its Complications; Part 1: Diagnosis and Classification of Diabetes Mellitus. Department of Non communicable Disease Surveillance, Geneva, 1999.

155. MacPherson H, Altman DG, Hammerschlag R, Youping L, Taixiang W, et al. (2010) . Revised STandards for Reporting Interventions in Clinical Trials of Acupuncture (STRICTA): Extending the CONSORT Statement. PLoS Medicine, 7(6), pp. 1-11

156. Berger, V. W. & Alperson, S. Y., 2009. A General Framework for the Evaluation of Clinical Trial Quality. Reviews on Recent Clinical Trials, 4(2), pp. 79-88.

157. ZHAO Hui-ling, GAO Xin , GAO Yan-bin , et al. Clinical Observation on Effect of Acupuncture in Treating Diabetic Peripheral Neuropathy . Chinese Journal of Integrated Traditional and Western Medicine (C JITWM) in April 2007 Volume 27 No. 4 C JITWM, April 2007, Vol.21, No.4 (312-314).

158. Role of acupuncture in the management of diabetic painful neuropathy (DPN): a pilot RCT. Garrow AP, Xing M, Vere J, Verrall B, Wang L, Jude EB.Acupunct Med. 2014 Jun;32(3):242-9.

159. Acupuncture for distal symmetric multiple peripheral neuropathy of diabetes mellitus: a randomized controlled trial. Lu M, Li K, Wang J. Zhongguo Zhen Jiu. 2016 May; 36(5):481-4.

160. Clinical observation on diabetic peripheral neuropathy treated with electroacupuncture and acupoint injection. Jin Z, Zhang BF, Shang LX, Wang LN, Wang YL, Chen J, Jiang SS. Zhongguo Zhen Jiu. 2011 Jul; 31(7):613-6.

161. Effect of spleen-stomach regulation-needling on nerve conduction activity in patients with diabetic peripheral neuropathy. Ji XQ[1], Wang CM, Zhang P, Zhang X, Zhang ZL. Zhen Ci Yan Jiu. 2010 Dec; 35(6):443-7.

162. Fifteenday acupuncture treatment relieves diabetic peripheral neuropathy.Tong Y1, Guo H, Han B. J Acupunct Meridian Stud. 2010 Jun; 3(2):95-103. doi: 10.1016/S2005-2901(10)60018-0.

163. Clinical effects of acupuncture for diabetic peripheral neuropathy. Zhang C, Ma YX, Yan Y. J Tradit Chin Med. 2010 Mar; 30(1):13-4.

References

164. Effects of penetrating acupuncture on peripheral nerve conduction velocity in patients with diabetic peripheral neuropathy: a randomized controlled trial.Chen YL, Ma XM, Hou WG, Cen J, Yu XM, Zhang L. Zhong Xi Yi Jie He Xue Bao. 2009 Mar; 7(3):273-5.

165. Clinical study on the wrist-ankle acupuncture treatment for 30 cases of diabetic peripheral neuritis. Jiang H[1], Shi K, Li X, Zhou W, Cao Y. J Tradit Chin Med. 2006 Mar; 26(1):8-12.

166. Acupuncture Treatment of Diabetic Peripheral Neuropathy in an American Indian Community. Anne Bailey, Deborah Wingard, Matthew Allison, Priscilla Summers, Daniel Calac. J Acupunct Meridian Stud 2017; 10(2):90-95.

167. Clinical Observation of Warm Acupuncture in Treating Diabetic Peripheral Neuropathy. SUN Yuan-zheng, XU Ying-ying. J. Acupunct. Tuina. Sci. 2010, 8 (5): 287-290.

168. Wang Hui, Zhang Huijin, Wang Ping, Li Yinghong. Treatment of Diabetic Peripheral Neuropathy by Different Acupuncture Methods Comparison of clinical outcomes. Guiding Journal of Traditional Chinese Medicine and Pharmacy October.2015; Vol.21 No.19- (10-11).

169. Zhao Zhixuan 1, Liu Ting 1, Li Mo. Treatment of 48 Cases of Diabetic Peripheral Neuropathy with Scalp acupuncture. JCAM. Nov, 2010, Vol.26, NO.11- (6-8).

170. FEI Ai-hua, CAI Sheng-chao, CHEN Ying, ZHU Cai-feng, QIN Xiao-feng. Therapeutic Effect of Acupuncture on Diabetic Peripheral Neuropathy and Its Influence on hs-CRP. Shanghai J Acu-mox, Feb 2011, Vol 30, No 2- (99-100).

171. GAO Yu. The clinical effect of acupuncture and moxibustion in the treatment of diabetic peripheral neuropathy. Journal of Traditional Chinese Medicine, November 2016 (128-129)

172. ZUO Lin, ZHANG Lin. Study on the Effect of Acupuncture plus Methylcobalamin in Treating Diabetic Peripheral Neuropathy. J. Acupunct. Tuina. Sci. 2010, 8 (4): 249-252

173. The 1999 American Diabetes Association (ADA) diagnostic criteria for diagnosis of type 2 diabetes

174. Shen Xiaozhou. Chronic complications of diabetes. Shanghai: Shanghai Medical University Press, 1999: 206- 287.

175. Jiang Yuping. Clinical Neurological Diseases. Shanghai: Shanghai Medical University Press, 1999: 476- 486.

# References

176. Qian Zhaoren, Zhong Xueli. Diabetic Neuropathy. Shanghai Medical 1984; (7): 426-427.

177. Lin Lan.Chinese Journal of Traditional Chinese Medicine. Chinese Journal of Medicine 1998; (4): 3-4.

178.   Xiao T .Japanese diabetic polyneuropathy simple diagnostic criteria (2002 revision)[ S] . Zh ongguo Yi Xue Sheng Lu n T an Bao (Chin Med Stud T rib , Chin), 2002 , 5 :16

179. Revill SI, Robinson JO, Rosen M, Hogg MIJ (1976). The reliability of a linear analogue for evaluating pain. Anaesthesia 31: 1191–1198

180.  Ametov AS, Barinov A, Dyck PJ, Hermann R, Kozlova N, et al. (2003) The sensory symptoms of diabetic polyneuropathy are improved with alpha-lipoic: the SYDNEY trial. Diabetes Care 26: 770–776

181. Wei Chen, Guo-yan Yang, Bo Liu, Eric Manheimer and Jian-Ping Liu. Manual Acupuncture for Treatment of Diabetic Peripheral Neuropathy: A Systematic Review of Randomized Controlled Trials. PLOS, September 12, 2013.

182. Tang JL, Zhan SY, Ernst E (1999) Review of randomised controlled trials of traditional Chinese medicine. BMJ 319: 160–61.

183. Liu JP (2009) What should we do with the growing amount of TCM research published in the Chinese literature? Focus on Alternative and Complementary Therapies 14: 92–93.

184. Wenjing Xiong, Xue Feng, Jianping Liu, Wei Chen. Electroacupuncture for treatment of diabetic peripheral neuropathy: A systematic review of randomized controlled trials. Journal of Traditional Chinese Medical Sciences (2016) 3, 9-21

185. Chen Bo., Zhao Xue., Guo Yi, Chen Zelin, Bai Yang, Wang Zixu, Wang Yajun. Assessing the Quality of Reports about Randomized Controlled Trials of Acupuncture Treatment on Diabetic Peripheral Neuropathy.  PLoS ONE- www.plosone.org 1 July 2012 | Volume 7 | Issue 7 | e38461

186. Lu X, Hongcai S, Jiaying W, Jing H, Jun X (2011) Assessing the Quality of Reports about Randomized Controlled Trials of Acupuncture Treatment on Mild Cognitive Impairment. PLoS ONE 6(2): e16922.

187. Wu T, Li Y, Bian Z, Liu G, Moher D (2009) Randomized trials published in some Chinese journals: how many are randomized? Trials 10: 46

188. Haiyong Chen , Zhipeng Ning , Wing Lok Lam , et al. Types of Control in Acupuncture Clinical Trials Might Affect the Conclusion of the Trials: A Review of Acupuncture on Pain Management. J Acupunct Meridian Stud 2016;9(5):227-233.

References

189. Manheimer E (2011) Selecting a control for in vitro fertilization and acupuncture randomized controlled trials (RCTs): how sham controls may unnecessarily complicate the RCT evidence base. FertilSteril 95: 2456–2461.

190. Dimitrova A, Murchison C, Oken B. Acupuncture for the Treatment of Peripheral Neuropathy: A Systematic Review and Meta-Analysis. J Altern Complement Med. 2017 Mar; 23(3):164-179.

191. Higgins JPT, Altman DG, Sterne JAC (editors) (2011) Chapter 8: Assessing risk of bias in included studies. In: Higgins JPT, Green S (editors). Cochrane Handbook for Systematic Reviews of Interventions Version 5.1.0 (updated March 2011). The Cochrane Collaboration, 2011. Available from www.cochrane-handbook.org.

192. Melchart D, Weidenhammer W, Streng A, Reitmayr S, Hoppe A, et al. (2004) Prospective investigation of adverse effects of acupuncture in 97 733 patients. Arch Intern Med 164: 104–105.

193. Witt CM, Pach D, Brinkhaus B, Wruck K, Tag B, et al. (2009) Safety of acupuncture: results of a prospective observational study with 229,230 patients and introduction of a medical information and consent form. Forsch Komplementmed 16: 91–7.

194. MacPherson H, Thomas K, Walters S, Fitter M (2001) The York acupuncture safety study: prospective survey of 34 000 treatments by traditional acupuncturists. BMJ 323: 486–487.

195. White A, Hayhoe S, Hart A, Ernst E (2001) Adverse events following acupuncture: prospective survey of 32 000 consultations with doctors and physiotherapists. BMJ 323: 485–486.

196. Savović J, Jones HE, Altman DG, Harris RJ, Jüni P, et al. (2012) Influence of reported study design characteristics on intervention effect estimates from randomized, controlled trials. Ann Intern Med 157: 429–438.

197. Sun Y, Lai MS, Lu CJ (2005) Effectiveness of vitamin B12 on diabetic neuropathy: systematic review of clinical controlled trials. Acta Neurol Taiwan 14: 48–54.

198. Li J, Wan Z (2008) Prostaglandin E1 in conjunction with high doses of vitamin B12 improves nerve conduction velocity of patients with diabetic peripheral neuropathy. Neural Regeneration Research 3: 529–532.

The following are some of

*Dr. Samir Yousef Ahmed AbouHussein (The Author of this book)* international contributions during the year 2019.

# 16th Meeting of the Mediterranean Group for the Study of Diabetes

## Poster Prize

NORTH BANK

awarded to

### Samir ABOUHUSSEIN

in recognition of his contribution to the advancement
of knowledge in the field of diabetes mellitus.

Casablanca, April 12, 2019

*Prof. P. Conthe, MGSD President*

This prize is supported by a grant from      SERVIER

112

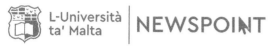

# International award for research from the UM Centre for Traditional Chinese Medicine

Newspoint (https://www.um.edu.mt/newspoint) > News (https://www.um.edu.mt/newspoint/news) > Features (https://www.um.edu.mt/newspoint/news/features) > 2019 (https://www.um.edu.mt/newspoint/news/features/2019) > May (https://www.um.edu.mt/newspoint/news/features/2019/05) > International award for research from the UM Centre for Traditional Chinese Medicine (https://www.um.edu.mt/newspoint/news/features/2019/05/internationalawardforresearchfromtheuniversitycentrefortraditionalchinesemedicine)

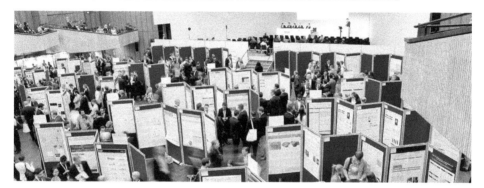

The Mediterranean Group for the Study of Diabetes during its biennial meeting held in Morocco in April 2019 has awarded Dr Samir Yousef Ahmed AbouHussein, a Master's graduate from the University of Malta Centre for Traditional Chinese Medicine, the prize for the best poster presented from the North Mediterranean (European) Bank.

Dr AbouHussein, a Palestinian medical doctor and researcher resident in Malta, has previously investigated the contribution the individual's genetic has towards contributing to the development of gestational diabetes in the Maltese population. The current research formed part of his Master's research thesis investigating the role of acupuncture techniques in the management of diabetic peripheral neuropathy.

Dr AbouHussein's meta-analysis showed that there appears to be a positive role for acupuncture treatment in the management of diabetic peripheral neuropathy, though further randomised controlled trials are necessary. The research follows the principles of investigating the role of integrative medicine in the management of different medical pathologies thus expanding the therapeutic tools of the contemporary practitioner.

Quicklinks ▾

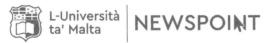

L-Università ta' Malta | **NEWSPOINT**

# Research presented at the 4th Mering Diabetes Technology & Prevention Symposium in Cottbus-Germany

Newspoint (https://www.um.edu.mt/newspoint) > News (https://www.um.edu.mt/newspoint/news) > Features (https://www.um.edu.mt/newspoint/news/features) > 2019 (https://www.um.edu.mt/newspoint/news/features/2019) > June (https://www.um.edu.mt/newspoint/news/features/2019/06) > Research presented at the 4th Mering Diabetes Technology & Prevention Symposium in Cottbus-Germany (https://www.um.edu.mt/newspoint/news/features/2019/06/researchpresentedatthe4thmeringdiabetestechnologyAndpreventionsymposiumincottbus-germany)

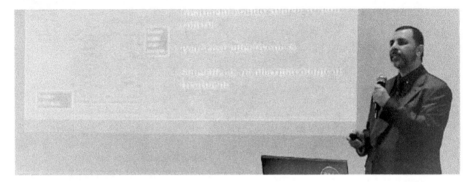

Research work on integrative medical systems, carried out by Dr Samir Yousef Ahmed AbouHussein, under the auspices of the Centre for Traditional Chinese Medicine (https://www.um.edu.mt/tcm), was presented at the annual 4th Mering Diabetes Technology & Prevention Symposium in Cottbus-Germany on 10 May 2019.

The work, carried out as part of the Master in Traditional Chinese Medicine degree, analysed the role of acupuncture as a complimentary management for diabetic peripheral neuropathy. The presentation was one of the three finalist submissions for the competitive Mering Research session 2019.

Quicklinks ▾

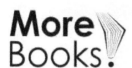
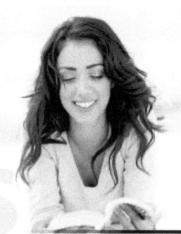
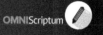

Lightning Source UK Ltd.
Milton Keynes UK
UKHW010754031022
409789UK00009B/5

9 786139 472253